Whispers Of The Womb

Healing Generations and Reclaiming Feminine Power

Sarmistha Mitra
Spiritual Psychologist
&
Holistic Health Expert

Whispers Of The Womb : Healing Generations and Reclaiming Feminine Power is a non-fiction work intended for informational and educational purposes.

The insights, examples, and narratives presented are based on research, professional experience, and real-life observations. While care has been taken to ensure accuracy, some details may have been adapted or anonymized to protect individual privacy. Any resemblance to specific individuals, events, or entities is unintentional and coincidental. The book does not substitute professional advice; readers are encouraged to seek appropriate support for their personal circumstances.

All rights reserved. No part of this book may be reproduced in any form or by any electronic or mechanical means, including information storage and retrieval systems, without written permission from the author, except by a reviewer who may quote passages for a review.

©AllCopyright 2025 Sarmistha Mitra
First Edition: 2025

Table of Contents

Title Page

Copyright

Dedication

Epigraph

Contents

Introduction: Listening to the whispers of the womb.

Chapter 1: Understanding the Whispers of the Womb

Chapter 2: The Ancestral Imprints in the Womb

Chapter 3: Recognizing Physical Manifestations of Womb Imbalances

Chapter 4: Releasing Emotional Trauma Stored in the Womb

Chapter 5: Reclaiming Your Feminine Power Through Subconscious Reprogramming

Chapter 6: Healing Generational Inadequacies and Breaking Cycles

Chapter 7: Integrating Womb Healing with Energy Practices

Chapter 8: Reconnecting with Creative and Sexual Energy

Chapter 9: Womb Healing Practices for Physical Wellness

Chapter 10: Living with the Empowered Womb

Bonus Section: Practical Resources and Tools for Ongoing Womb Healing

Appendices

Conclusion: Embracing a Life of Wholeness and Worth

About The Author

Books By This Author

With profound gratitude, I extend my heartfelt thanks to those who have been part of my journey—those who have walked beside me in this path of healing, discovery, and transformation.

To my family, your unwavering support has been the foundation upon which I have built my understanding of deep inner work. Your encouragement has given me the strength to delve into the depths of my soul, unraveling the complexities of the human experience, and for that, I am eternally grateful.

To my readers; this book is a tribute to your resilience, to your openness, and to the unwavering belief in the sacred potential of transformation; you are the true inspiration behind this book. May this work serve as a beacon of hope, a sanctuary of wisdom, and a guide for those who walk the path of womb healing and self-discovery. Thank you for trusting me to be a small part of your journey.

Beloved Readers,

I have devoted my life to exploring the mysteries of the human mind and understanding how our subconscious beliefs shape every aspect of our lives. Through years of work, I have witnessed the profound connection between the mind, body, and spirit—particularly in women's health.

Today, I want to share a deeply personal reflection that has shaped my understanding of womb health and its complex interplay with energy, societal expectations, and ancestral imprints.

This realization began within my own family. One of my first encounters with womb-related challenges was with my aunt, who faced the immense pain of being unable to bear children. Her journey was marked by emotional anguish, societal judgment, and an unbearable weight of unmet expectations. I then watched my cousin sister endure years of IVF treatments in her effort to conceive. While she eventually succeeded, the intensive hormonal treatments left her with lasting physical damage. Witnessing their struggles opened my eyes to how deeply our societal conditioning and physical health are intertwined, especially in the sacred space of the womb.

As I stepped into my role as a counselor, my understanding deepened further. My very first client was also a woman grappling with infertility. She was undergoing IVF treatments, exhausted and emotionally drained, when she came across information about subconscious reprogramming and sought my help. During our sessions, we began to unearth her inner resistance and deeply buried subconscious beliefs—feelings of inadequacy, fear of failure, and layers of unhealed ancestral trauma that were deeply rooted within her. By working together to recognize and release these blocks, she experienced a profound shift. Shortly after, she conceived naturally—a moment that affirmed the power of addressing the mind-body connection.

These experiences led me to ask deeper questions:
Why are womb-related diseases and infertility on the rise today?
What has shifted within women's lives that is contributing to this imbalance?

In my search for answers, I saw how women have shifted into predominantly masculine roles to meet societal demands—to be assertive, driven, and constantly "on." While these traits are undeniably valuable, this overemphasis on masculine energy is often a trauma response—a way to rebel against the confines of stereotypes, take back control, and assert their power. The desire to prove oneself, to be seen as good enough, capable, and worthy, can drive women to push themselves relentlessly. In doing so, many become disconnected from their natural feminine rhythms and suppress their true essence.

Statistics support this theory and highlight the broader societal patterns at play. Fertility rates and womb-related disorders, such as uterine fibroid and endometriosis, reveal stark differences across socioeconomic and social strata:

Higher Socioeconomic Status (SES) and Fertility Issues: Women in higher SES brackets often experience delayed childbearing due to career demands, which can contribute to fertility challenges and higher rates of endometriosis. A study in the UK found that women in higher SES groups report more fertility problems, potentially linked to lifestyle factors and the stress of meeting societal and professional expectations. The constant drive for success can keep their bodies in a state of chronic stress, disrupting hormonal balance and manifesting in womb-related health issues.

Uterine Fibroids Among Minority Women: Black women, in particular, experience a significantly higher prevalence of uterine fibroids. Studies indicate that among asymptomatic women aged 18–30, 25.5% of Black women had fibroids, compared to 6.9% of White women. This disparity may be influenced by genetic predispositions but also by stress, societal pressures, and environmental factors. The chronic stress of navigating a world marked by discrimination and unique cultural challenges can exacerbate health issues and reflect deeper energetic imbalances.

Lower Socioeconomic Status and Fertility Rates: Women from lower SES backgrounds often have higher fertility rates, driven by different societal norms, reduced access to contraceptive methods, and varying healthcare availability. However, they may face fewer womb-related disorders due to closer ties to traditional roles, physical activity, and different environmental exposures, providing a complex contrast to their higher SES counterparts.

The statistics and observations validate a critical aspect of my theory: the imbalance in the body's rhythm, especially within the womb, is heavily influenced by societal pressures, the drive to prove oneself, and the disruption of feminine energy. High expectations, societal norms, and the need for constant validation often place women in a chronic state of stress, causing an over-stimulation of their autonomic nervous system and disrupting their natural rhythms. The suppression of feminine energy and the overuse of masculine traits can lead to disconnection and physical manifestations of imbalance within the womb space.

This constant drive and need for validation

often leave the body in a state of high alert, with the autonomic nervous system (ANS) stuck in survival mode. The fight, flight, or freeze response becomes a constant companion, disrupting the body's natural rhythms and creating an environment where womb-related imbalances can manifest. Hormonal disruptions, chronic stress, and suppressed emotions all take their toll on the feminine center—the womb.

But the imbalance goes even deeper. For many women, there is also the weight of inherited trauma—generational pain and beliefs passed down from ancestors who faced suppression, control, and unhealed wounds. These epigenetic memories are often stored in the womb space, creating subconscious patterns that influence physical health and emotional well-being.

Healing, therefore, involves more than just addressing physical symptoms; it requires a holistic approach that balances masculine and feminine energies, releases subconscious resistance, and honors the power and sacredness of the womb.

Healing requires more than physical treatments. It demands a holistic approach to restoring balance, addressing subconscious resistance to dominance or submission, restoring harmony by reconnecting with the feminine energy within.

This involves releasing inherited trauma, recognizing the societal pressures we face, and embracing our true selves without the need for constant validation. Only then can women find harmony, reclaim their power, and experience profound healing in their body and spirit.

In working with clients, I have seen the power of reconnecting with our true selves, of allowing the feminine energy to flow freely once more. It is a journey of transformation, of shifting from survival to thriving, from imbalance to harmony. By understanding the root causes of these imbalances—societal pressures, energetic misalignment, and inherited trauma—women can reclaim their health, their rhythm, and their power.

This is the path I have dedicated my life to guiding others on, and it is an honor to share this journey of healing and empowerment with each of you. Together, we can break free from the cycles of imbalance and return to the wholeness that lies within us all.

Introduction: Listening to the whispers of the womb.

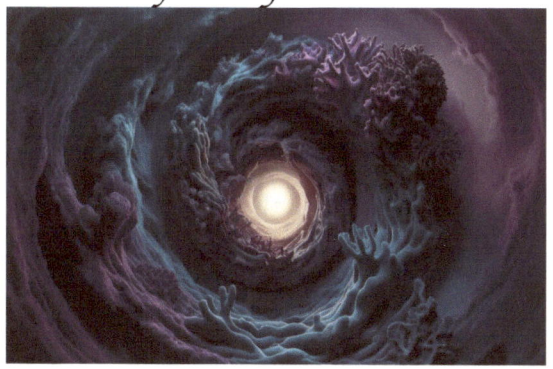

The womb represents the core of feminine energy—a profound center of creation, intuition, and power. When you learn to listen to the Whispers of the womb, you realize that healing is the journey of reconnecting with this sacred space, unraveling layers of unhealed trauma, inherited beliefs, and societal conditioning that have silenced or suppressed the feminine essence. In my work with women, I've observed that the womb carries emotional imprints, generational memories, and societal narratives that have long shaped the female experience. Womb healing isn't just a physical restoration but a holistic reclamation of one's identity, self-worth, and potential.

Defining Womb Healing

At its heart, womb healing is about reconnecting with the feminine essence that resides within each woman. This isn't just about physical healing but a reawakening of the *shakti*, or feminine power, that the womb symbolizes. In many cultures, the womb is revered as the seat of creation—a place not only of physical birth but also of emotional and spiritual regeneration. When we heal our wombs, we access a deeper part of ourselves that holds our intuition, creativity, and ability to nurture ourselves and others.

The womb's energy is often associated with the sacral chakra, which governs our emotions, relationships, and creative energies. Just as the mind is a repository for thoughts, beliefs, and memories, the womb holds a unique archive of experiences. These experiences can be deeply personal—stemming from trauma, relationships, and personal beliefs—or ancestral, inherited from generations of women before us. When we embark on womb healing, we're essentially peeling back these layers, honoring the stories they carry, and releasing what no longer serves us.

Cultural Significance of the Womb in Ancient and Modern Societies

Throughout history, the womb has been revered and symbolized as the ultimate source of life, creativity, and feminine power. In many ancient cultures, the feminine essence rooted in the womb was seen as sacred and central to societal balance. However, as patriarchal structures took hold, this reverence shifted, leading to the suppression of women's roles, autonomy, and connection to their wombs.

Ancient Societies and the Womb's Sacredness

In ancient matriarchal societies, such as those found in pre-patriarchal Europe and various Indigenous cultures worldwide, the womb was celebrated as a symbol of life and renewal. Goddesses like Isis of Ancient Egypt, Demeter of Greece, and Shakti in Hinduism represented fertility, creation, and the cyclical nature of life. Rituals and ceremonies often centered around the cycles of menstruation, birth, and rebirth, reflecting a deep understanding of women's connection to nature and the cosmos.

The Red Tent Tradition: In some ancient cultures, menstruating women would retreat to a "red tent" or a sacred space, where they would rest, reflect, and bond with other women. This time of retreat recognized the inherent power of the womb and allowed women to honor their cycles. It was a communal acknowledgment of their ability to create life, both physically and metaphorically.

The Moon Cycles and Womb Wisdom: Many Indigenous traditions linked the cycles of the womb with the moon's phases, recognizing a powerful connection between a woman's body and the rhythms of nature. The waxing and waning of the moon mirrored women's cyclical nature, with rituals and practices designed to harness this energy for creation, healing, and transformation.

The Shift to Patriarchal Structures and Women's Subordination

Over time, patriarchal systems emerged and gained dominance, leading to a systematic attempt to control and dominate women's bodies. Among patriarchs, the violation of the womb became a deliberate means of asserting power and control. During wartime, conquering soldiers often raped women of the enemy as a tactic of terror, domination, and subjugation. This heinous act was intended not only to physically harm women but also to break the spirit of entire communities, asserting control over the physical and generational lineage of their enemies.

In patriarchal societies, rape has also been used as a broader societal tool to strip women of their power, autonomy, and dignity. By assaulting women's bodies, patriarchal forces sought to demonstrate dominance and keep women in a state of fear, subordination, and disconnection from their power.

Modern Shifts and Feminine Reclamation

In more recent history, the feminist movement and a collective desire for women to reclaim autonomy over their bodies have led to a resurgence of interest in womb healing and feminine empowerment. Women are once again recognizing the sacredness of their wombs and seeking ways to reconnect with their inner power.

Rising Interest in Holistic Practices: The global rise of yoga, meditation, and holistic healing has sparked a renewed focus on the sacral chakra and womb energy. Practices like yoni steaming, womb meditation, and menstrual cycle awareness have empowered women to reconnect with their bodies, honor their cycles, and reclaim their feminine energy.

Women in Leadership and Balance: As women have entered the workforce and leadership roles, there has been a cultural shift in redefining what it means to embody feminine energy. While patriarchal structures still exist, modern women are finding ways to integrate their innate nurturing, intuitive, and creative qualities with assertive, goal-driven traits. This balance is part of a broader movement to heal historical wounds and imbalances inflicted upon the feminine essence.

Societal Roles, Cultural Imprints and the Impact on Women's Health

Historically, societal expectations have relegated women to roles of service, submission, and silence, shaping the ways they perceive themselves and their worth. The suppression of feminine energy over centuries has left deep imprints on women's health and well-being. Emotional repression, societal control, and the cultural narrative of shame surrounding menstruation, sexuality, and childbirth have led to disconnection from the womb and feelings of inadequacy, shame, and powerlessness. This historical suppression often manifests as womb-related disorders, from PCOS and endometriosis to infertility and fibroids, reflecting the physical manifestation of these cultural wounds. This cultural backdrop has left imprints on women's health and well-being. The suppression of feminine expression and the lack of autonomy over one's body have contributed to a range of psychological and physical health issues. Studies have shown that emotional repression can lead to stress and hormonal imbalances, affecting reproductive health (Gabor Maté, *When the*

Body Says No). Moreover, the constant need to meet imposed expectations creates emotional strain, which accumulates within the body, particularly in the womb.

The womb, as an organ and an energy center, carries these unspoken pains and unacknowledged burdens.

It's no coincidence that modern women face an epidemic of womb-related disorders, from PCOS and endometriosis to infertility and fibroids. These physical conditions are often intertwined with deep-seated feelings of inadequacy, shame, and powerlessness, reflective of the societal neglect and disempowerment women have historically faced. As we address these conditions from a holistic perspective, it becomes clear that healing the womb is also a journey of restoring feminine identity and self-worth.

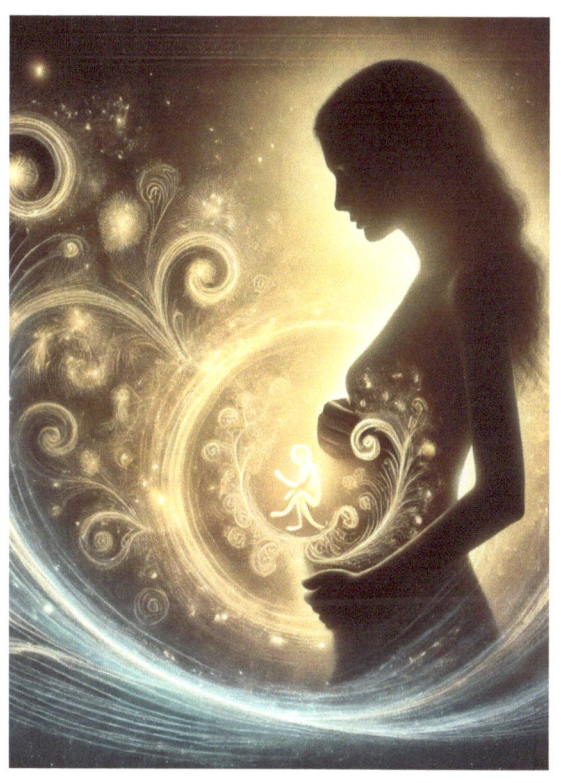

Generational and Ancestral Imprints in the Womb

Our wombs carry not only our personal stories but also the imprints of our ancestral lineage. Just as we inherit physical traits, we inherit emotional and psychological patterns. Epigenetic research indicates that trauma experienced by one generation can alter the genetic expression in subsequent generations (Yehuda & Bierer, *Biological Psychiatry*). This means that unresolved traumas—such as feelings of inadequacy, shame, or oppression—can be passed down, residing in the bodies of descendants. These generational imprints manifest as subconscious beliefs, fears, or even physical symptoms. Women may feel inexplicable shame, a fear of being "not enough," or a deep-seated sense of worthlessness, without realizing that these feelings are echoes of their ancestors' experiences. Womb healing is a way to honor these stories, acknowledge the pain carried through generations, and consciously release it. By doing so, we free not only ourselves but also future generations from repeating these cycles.

In my *DecodeYou®* approach, I often guide women through practices to recognize and release these ancestral patterns. By accessing these imprints within the subconscious mind and body, women can heal inherited wounds, transforming feelings of inadequacy into empowerment and reclaiming their own unique potential. This is a form of liberation that goes beyond personal healing—it is a gift to one's lineage and a step toward healing collective feminine wounds.

The Benefits of Womb Healing

Womb healing offers a multi-dimensional approach to wellness that touches every aspect of a woman's life. Here's how:

1. Emotional Freedom: Releasing unresolved emotions held within the womb allows women to experience greater emotional clarity and balance. This healing process sheds light on patterns of self-sabotage, fear, and unworthiness, liberating women from subconscious cycles that have kept them from living authentically.

2. Physical Wellness: By addressing the emotional and energetic causes of womb-related conditions, women can experience physical relief from symptoms like menstrual pain, hormonal imbalances, and reproductive issues. Studies support the idea that emotional release can have positive effects on physical health, as unresolved stress and trauma often manifest in the body (Candace Pert, *Molecules of Emotion*). Womb healing, therefore, provides a pathway to restoring physical harmony.

3. Spiritual Awakening: The womb is often referred to as a portal for creation and spiritual insight. When women connect with their wombs, they access a deep well of intuition, creativity, and inner wisdom.

This connection enables them to live with greater purpose, align with their true selves, and engage with life from a place of wholeness.

4. Generational Release: Healing the womb allows women to break generational cycles of trauma and disempowerment. By releasing the inherited beliefs and patterns stored in the womb, they not only heal themselves but also free their lineage from these burdens. This generational release brings a renewed sense of freedom, empowering future generations to live without the weight of unhealed ancestral pain.

Womb healing is a journey I wholeheartedly recommend to all women. It is not only a deeply personal journey but also a transformative process that holds the potential to create broader societal harmony, where men and women stand together—not in dominance or submission but in balance, mutual respect, and true partnership. Here's why this aspect is essential and how womb healing contributes to it:

1. Healing Gender-Based Trauma and Restoring Balance

Historically, patriarchy has enforced systems of dominance and control that have led to the suppression of feminine energy and, in turn, wounded masculine energy. This imbalance has created cycles of dominance and submission, leading to emotional, social, and relational disharmony. Womb healing invites women to reclaim their power, and by doing so, it encourages men to reconnect with their own authentic selves, fostering healthier dynamics based on mutual respect.

When women heal the wounds carried within their wombs—wounds of suppression, shame, and inherited trauma—

they contribute to a collective rebalancing of energies, allowing both men and women to relate to each other from a place of wholeness and equality.

2. Dissolving the Patterns of Dominance and Submission

The act of womb healing is about more than individual empowerment; it is about breaking free from the deeply rooted patterns of dominance and submission that have defined gender relations for centuries. When women embody their true feminine essence without the need to prove, submit, or dominate, they create space for men to step into their authentic selves without fear of overpowering or being overpowered. This rebalancing allows for healthier, more authentic relationships—where neither gender seeks to dominate but rather to support, honor, and uplift each other. In this dynamic, men and women can co-create spaces of harmony, trust, and shared purpose.

3. Encouraging Empathy, Compassion, and Understanding

As women undergo the journey of womb healing, they cultivate greater self-awareness, empathy, and compassion—qualities that naturally extend outward into their relationships and interactions with others. This encourages men to do the same, creating a ripple effect of empathy and understanding that bridges the divide between genders. It leads to deeper connections and the dissolution of harmful stereotypes and power imbalances.

harmony. When women embrace and heal their sacred feminine energy, and men honor and balance their own masculine energy, they co-create a world where each individual's gifts are valued and celebrated. Together, we can build a society that thrives on collaboration, compassion, and equality, creating a better future for all.

Chapter 1: Understanding the Whispers of the Womb

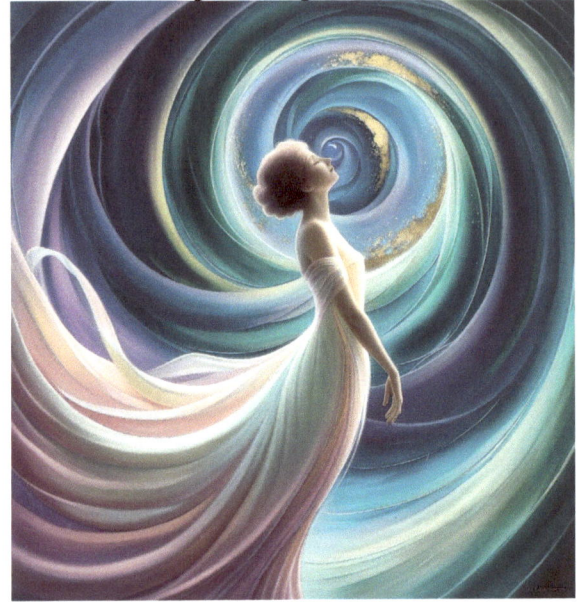

The womb is far more than a reproductive organ; it is a profound center of life, creativity, intuition, and connection within the female body.

Both energetically and physiologically, the womb holds immense power and significance, symbolizing the wellspring of feminine strength, wisdom, and intuition. To understand the whispers of the womb is to recognize it as a vessel for not only physical creation but also for deep emotional, spiritual, and energetic connection.

The Energetic and Physiological Significance of the Womb

Physiologically, the womb provides the space for nurturing and sustaining new life. This capacity for creation underscores one of humanity's most powerful potentials: the ability to bring life into the world. However, the womb's significance extends far beyond its reproductive function. It is sensitive to hormonal fluctuations, making it deeply connected to a woman's emotional and psychological states.

The womb also serves as an energetic center, storing life experiences, emotional memories, and even generational imprints.

This concept has roots in ancient wisdom, where the womb was revered as a sacred vessel—a repository of feminine power, intuition, and the deepest truths of life. In modern times, the connection between emotions and physical health has been substantiated by researchers like Dr. Candace Pert, who demonstrated that emotions influence cellular memory and manifest within the body. Just as unprocessed trauma can affect the heart or muscles, the womb uniquely absorbs and reflects unresolved emotions and generational traumas. Therefore, healing the womb is not just about restoring physical health; it is a holistic process of releasing stored emotional burdens and cultivating harmony within.

The Womb as a Center of Creativity, Intuition, and Nurturing

The womb's capacity for creation goes beyond physical birth; it is a source of creativity and inspiration. Many traditions view creativity as an extension of life force energy, and for women, the womb serves as a direct link to this energy. By connecting with the womb, women tap into an inner wellspring of creative potential, influencing all areas of life, from relationships to personal endeavors and artistic pursuits. This creative force drives our dreams, visions, and passions, making the womb a central aspect of self-expression.

The womb is also intimately connected with intuition. Often referred to as "gut feeling" or "inner knowing," this intuitive wisdom is deeply rooted in the body. When we tune into the womb, we access an instinctive guidance that transcends rational thought. It serves as a repository for unexpressed emotions—grief, joy, longing, love—and influences how we perceive and respond to life. This connection to emotional depth highlights why practices focused on the womb often lead to profound healing and self-awareness.

The nurturing aspect of the womb mirrors its physical role. Just as it nurtures life, it also nurtures our inner emotional landscape, providing a safe space to process, heal, and transform. Womb-centered practices such as meditation, visualization, and body-centered therapies can lead to emotional release and greater compassion, empathy, and self-love. Women who connect with their wombs often report feeling renewed and empowered, allowing them to nurture themselves and their relationships authentically.

The Connection between the Sacral Chakra and the Womb

In energy healing systems, especially in the yogic tradition, the womb is associated with the sacral chakra, or Swadhisthana, located below the navel. This chakra governs creativity, sexuality, pleasure, and emotional expression, serving as a focal point for identity and how we relate to the world. When energy flows freely through the sacral chakra, women experience emotional resilience, vibrant creativity, and balanced reproductive health. Conversely, blockages—often caused by trauma, suppressed emotions, or limiting beliefs—can lead to imbalances, manifesting as reproductive issues, creative stagnation, or emotional disconnection.

Balancing and clearing the sacral chakra can restore energetic flow to the womb, allowing women to access greater emotional release, creativity, and vitality. Practices like meditation, breathwork, and visualization help to heal this chakra, reconnecting women with their sensuality, intuition, and joy. Womb healing is, in essence, a journey of sacral chakra healing that transforms how we experience ourselves, our bodies, and our relationships. Healing the sacral chakra also reshapes our relationship with ourselves and others. A balanced sacral chakra fosters healthy boundaries, emotional clarity, and meaningful connections. By addressing these energies, women can break free from limiting narratives imposed by societal and personal experiences, realigning with a sense of self-worth and authenticity.

Summary: Chapter 1
To understand the sacred nature of the womb is to appreciate its role as more than a physical organ. It is a seat of creativity, intuition, emotional depth, and nurturing—

a space where life's deepest energies are cultivated and expressed. The connection between the womb and the sacral chakra further emphasizes its influence on how we relate to our bodies, emotions, and the world around us.

Womb healing is not merely about alleviating physical or emotional symptoms; it is a profound journey of reclaiming feminine power, wisdom, and self-love. By reconnecting with this sacred space, women unlock a source of intuitive knowing, creative inspiration, and nurturing potential that fuels every aspect of their lives. This process allows for deeper self-understanding, balance, and the cultivation of meaningful connections within and beyond oneself.

Chapter 2: The Ancestral Imprints in the Womb

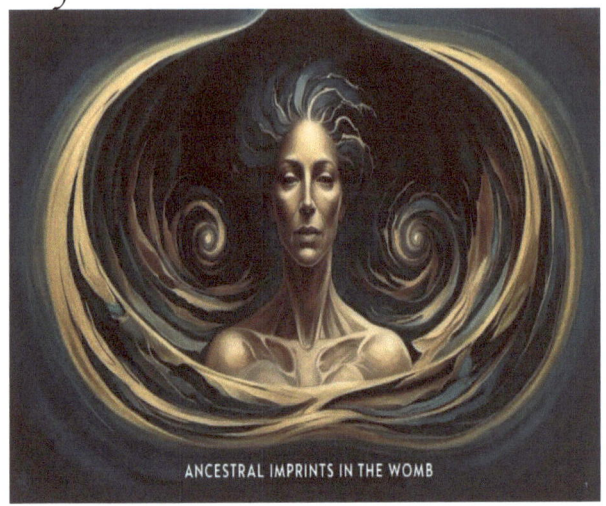

ANCESTRAL IMPRINTS IN THE WOMB

The womb is not only a physical and energetic center of creation but also a repository of inherited memories, emotions, and traumas. Just as physical traits are passed down from one generation to the next, so are emotional experiences and societal conditioning. This concept, often called *inherited trauma*, helps explain why some of the emotional, mental, and even physical patterns we experience may not originate solely from our personal lives—they are imprints from our ancestors. Understanding and healing these ancestral imprints within the womb is a powerful step toward reclaiming autonomy, health, and self-worth.

Inherited Trauma: A Legacy Carried in the Womb

The idea that trauma and emotional experiences are passed down through generations is supported by the field of epigenetics. Researchers have shown that trauma experienced by one generation can affect gene expression in subsequent generations. This alteration doesn't change the DNA structure itself but influences how genes are expressed, affecting physiological and emotional responses to stress (Yehuda & Bierer, *Biological Psychiatry*). For example, children and grandchildren of

Holocaust survivors have been found to carry higher stress hormone levels, showing physiological effects of their ancestors' trauma.

For women, the womb often becomes a repository for these inherited imprints. Emotions such as shame, fear, and inadequacy—feelings that previous generations may have repressed or left unresolved—are stored in this sacred space, influencing a woman's perception of herself and her role in the world. These inherited beliefs and emotions become "generational stories" that reside in our bodies and subconscious minds. When left unprocessed, they perpetuate cycles of pain and disempowerment until they are consciously identified and healed.

Each generation that does not process or heal these emotions unintentionally passes them along, creating a cycle that persists until it is consciously broken.

Manifestation of Ancestral Imprints as Womb-Related Conditions

When ancestral imprints remain unaddressed, they can manifest physically, often presenting as womb-related conditions. While these conditions have various contributing factors, unresolved trauma and inherited beliefs often play a significant role in creating an environment conducive to their development.

1. **PCOS (Polycystic Ovary Syndrome)**: PCOS, characterized by hormonal imbalances and irregular menstrual cycles, often signals a disconnection from the feminine cycle and self-worth. Generational beliefs surrounding women's roles, suppressed feminine expression, or feelings of inadequacy can contribute to this condition.

Women with ancestors who felt restricted, undervalued, or constrained may unconsciously carry shame or discomfort about their femininity, impacting hormonal health.

2. **Endometriosis**: This condition, marked by the growth of uterine tissue outside the womb, often reflects deep-seated pain or unresolved emotional suffering. Women with endometriosis may carry generational stories of hardship, shame, or feeling "out of place" in their own bodies or roles. This displacement and emotional pain can be manifestations of inherited trauma, with unresolved emotions becoming lodged in the womb and creating cycles of physical and emotional suffering.

3. **Infertility**: Infertility can reflect a subconscious block or resistance to the role of motherhood, possibly rooted in ancestral beliefs. For instance, women with

ancestors who faced oppression, trauma, or shame related to childbearing may carry subconscious fears or resistances tied to motherhood. This inherited fear or resistance can create blocks in the womb, impacting fertility on an emotional and, ultimately, physical level.

While these conditions have many contributing factors, the presence of ancestral imprints plays a significant role in creating an environment within the body that can lead to womb-related health issues. By healing these inherited traumas, women can help alleviate not only their own pain but also end the cycle for future generations.

Reflection Exercises to Identify Ancestral Stories of Inadequacy, Shame, or Imposed Roles

To begin the process of healing ancestral trauma, it is essential to understand and release the inherited beliefs and emotions stored within the womb. These exercises will guide you through connecting with the stories passed down from your lineage, identifying patterns of inadequacy, shame, or imposed roles that may be influencing your life.

Exercise 1: Tracing Ancestral Patterns Through Reflection

Find a Quiet Space: Sit comfortably in a space where you won't be disturbed. Take a few deep breaths to center yourself, allowing any tension in your body to melt away.

Visualize Your Ancestral Line: In your mind's eye, picture a line of women standing behind you—your mother, grandmother, great-grandmother, and all the women who came before them. Imagine these women, regardless of whether you knew them, as bearers of stories, beliefs, and experiences that have shaped your lineage.

Ask for Insight: Silently ask these women to share with you any feelings, stories, or beliefs that may have been passed down to you. You might ask questions like:

➢ "What unresolved emotions or beliefs have I inherited from you?"

➢ "What stories of inadequacy or shame do I carry on your behalf?"

➢ "How did societal expectations shape your life and affect how you felt about yourself?"

Listen and Reflect: Allow yourself to receive whatever comes up. You may sense a particular emotion, see an image, or have a memory surface. Trust whatever you experience, even if it seems vague or abstract.

Journal: Afterward, take a few minutes to write down any insights, memories, or emotions that came up. This exercise helps uncover generational stories and identifies the beliefs that may be affecting you subconsciously.

Exercise 2: Womb Meditation to Release Ancestral Imprints

Place Your Hands on Your Womb: Close your eyes and place your hands over your lower abdomen, bringing awareness to this sacred space. Feel the warmth and connection between your hands and your womb.

Breathe into the Womb: Take slow, deep breaths, directing each inhale into your womb. Imagine that with each breath, you're filling your womb with healing light and warmth.

Connect with Ancestral Pain: Visualize any pain, shame, or inadequacy you may carry within your womb as a dark cloud or shadowy form. Imagine this shadow representing the unhealed emotions of your ancestors.

Offer Compassion and Release: As you exhale, imagine sending warmth and compassion to this shadow. See it slowly dissolving, being released from your womb. Affirm silently, "I release all inherited pain and shame from my womb," or "I let go of the stories that no longer serve me."

Envision Light Filling the Space: As the shadow dissipates, imagine a beautiful, golden or orange light filling your womb, representing healing and freedom. Picture this light expanding, connecting you to a sense of peace and empowerment.

Close with Gratitude: Take a few moments to thank your ancestors for the lessons they've imparted, and acknowledge the healing taking place within you.

Exercise 3: Identifying Patterns of Inadequacy or Imposed Roles

Reflect on Family Stories: Take time to think about the stories you've heard from or about the women in your family. Consider questions like:

Were they encouraged or discouraged from pursuing their dreams?

How did they feel about their roles as mothers, daughters, or wives?

Did they experience any societal limitations or expectations that shaped their lives?

Recognize Patterns: Look for any recurring themes or patterns of inadequacy, shame, or restricted roles. For example, you might realize that the women in your family were often taught to put others' needs before their own or were expected to conform to traditional roles regardless of their personal aspirations.

Acknowledge Your Connection: Notice if these patterns resonate with your own experiences or beliefs. Write down any emotions or realizations that come up, acknowledging how these patterns may have influenced you.

Affirm Release: Use affirmations to release any beliefs that no longer serve you. Examples include:

"I release all inherited feelings of inadequacy."

"I honor my ancestors by embracing my own worth and power."

"I am free to define my own identity and role."

Summary: Chapter 2

The womb holds stories far older than our own experiences. Through these exercises, we recognize that some of the challenges and beliefs we face today are not only our own but have been carried through generations. As we identify and release these ancestral imprints, we honor our lineage while choosing to break free from cycles that no longer serve us.

By healing the ancestral pain stored in our wombs, we reclaim our freedom, health, and self-worth. This liberation creates a ripple effect, ensuring that we not only heal ourselves but also offer a healthier, more empowered foundation for future generations. The process of womb healing is both an act of self-love and an act of love for the women who came before and those yet to come.

Chapter 3: Recognizing Physical Manifestations of Womb Imbalances

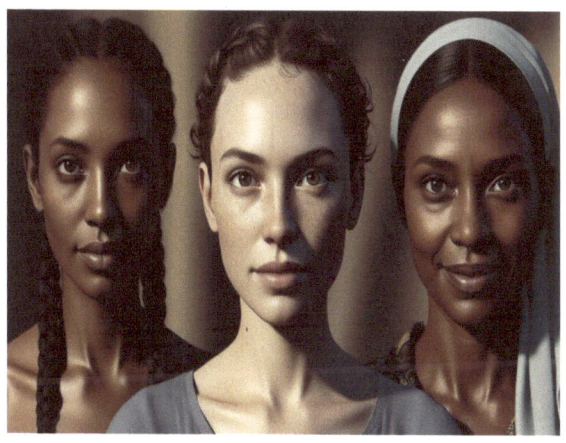

The womb holds not only the potential for life but also the accumulated stories, emotions, and experiences of a woman's lifetime and those of her lineage. Unprocessed trauma, suppressed emotions, and generational patterns often manifest in the womb, leading to physical conditions that carry deeper meanings. Understanding how these energies affect physical health opens the door to holistic healing, inviting us to address both the body and the subconscious mind.

How Trauma, Suppressed Emotions, and Generational Patterns Manifest in the Womb

The womb is highly sensitive to emotional energy. Just as muscles tighten in response to stress, the womb can absorb and store emotional pain, trauma, and unresolved memories. Traumas such as heartbreak, betrayal, abandonment, or feelings of inadequacy don't just disappear; they often reside in the body, becoming stored in areas like the womb where they subtly influence health. Even if these memories fade from conscious thought, their impact remains, creating energetic blockages that disrupt the natural flow of vitality in the womb space. Suppressed emotions can also affect the womb. Many women are conditioned to suppress emotions like anger, grief, or frustration, especially regarding issues related to their bodies or identities. These emotions, when unexpressed, settle within the womb, leading to physical and energetic imbalances. Over time, the stored energy builds up and can manifest as pain, irregularities, or reproductive health issues. Generational patterns play an equally significant role. Recent studies in epigenetics reveal that trauma can alter gene expression, affecting not just the individual but also their descendants (Yehuda & Bierer, *Biological Psychiatry*). Women may carry emotional patterns passed down through generations, such as fear, shame, or inadequacy, that affect the womb's physical and energetic health. These inherited patterns are often subconscious, yet they influence how women experience their bodies, relationships, and sense of worth.

Common Womb-Related Conditions and Their Emotional and Spiritual Underpinnings

Certain womb-related conditions frequently point to underlying emotional and spiritual blockages. While these conditions have medical explanations, exploring their emotional underpinnings offers a holistic path to healing, addressing the root causes that may be influencing physical symptoms.

1. Polycystic Ovary Syndrome (PCOS)

Medical Aspect: PCOS is a hormonal disorder that affects the ovaries, leading to irregular periods, cyst formation, and sometimes fertility challenges. It's associated with insulin resistance, weight gain, and elevated levels of androgens.

Emotional and Spiritual Underpinnings: PCOS is often linked to suppressed feminine energy. Women with PCOS may experience a disconnection from their femininity, feeling compelled to embrace masculine traits for survival or success. This condition may reflect internalized beliefs about the inadequacy of the feminine or fears of expressing vulnerability. Healing PCOS can involve reconnecting with the body, embracing femininity, and releasing beliefs that hinder a balanced expression of gendered energy.

2. Uterine Fibroids

Medical Aspect: Fibroids are noncancerous growths in the uterus, often causing heavy menstrual bleeding, pelvic pain, and complications with pregnancy.

Emotional and Spiritual Underpinnings: Fibroids are commonly associated with repressed anger, particularly anger tied to unmet needs, disappointments, or suppressed creative expression. Some traditions view fibroids as a physical manifestation of unexpressed creativity or unfulfilled desires. Women with fibroids may benefit from exploring where they feel stifled or unheard and practicing healthy ways to release suppressed emotions and pursue passions.

3. Menstrual Pain and Irregularities

Medical Aspect: Painful periods, irregular cycles, and conditions like endometriosis often involve inflammation, hormonal imbalances, and tissue growth outside the uterus.

Emotional and Spiritual Underpinnings: Menstrual pain can point to an internal conflict with one's feminine identity or negative beliefs about menstruation, sexuality, or womanhood. This condition may also reflect inherited patterns of shame or discomfort around femininity. Healing menstrual pain involves addressing both the physical and emotional body, cultivating self-acceptance, and releasing inherited beliefs about female cycles.

4. Infertility

Medical Aspect: Infertility has various physical causes, including hormonal imbalances, structural issues, and lifestyle factors, affecting a woman's ability to conceive.

Emotional and Spiritual Underpinnings: Infertility is often linked to deep-seated fears around motherhood, worthiness, or unresolved grief. Women may carry subconscious fears about bringing children into the world or feel unworthy of becoming mothers. Ancestral trauma, particularly involving loss, abandonment, or grief, can also play a role. Addressing these subconscious patterns can help release the emotional blocks associated with fertility.

5. Vaginal Dryness and the Loss of Feminine Flow

Emotional and Spiritual Aspects: Vaginal dryness, especially in premenopausal or even younger women, can be linked to stress, suppressed emotions, and disconnection from one's feminine energy. The vaginal tissues are extremely responsive to hormonal balance, which in turn is sensitive to stress levels, emotional states, and energy flow within the body. When a woman feels unsupported, pressured to perform, or disconnected from her feminine essence, her body may reflect this through dryness, a lack of lubrication, and even discomfort during intimacy.

Energetic Disconnection: Vaginal dryness may signify a disconnection from pleasure, sensuality, or the inability to relax and receive. In patriarchal societies, women's sexuality has often been controlled, suppressed, or shamed. The body may react by shutting down natural responses, leading to dryness and discomfort.

6. Inability to Reach Orgasm During Intercourse

Emotional and Spiritual Aspects: The inability to reach orgasm can be deeply tied to emotional, psychological, and even generational factors. Women who carry subconscious beliefs around shame, fear, or a lack of self-worth may find it difficult to fully surrender during intimacy. Orgasm requires trust, safety, and the ability to be present in one's body, which can be hindered by past trauma, societal conditioning, or inherited beliefs about sexuality.

Subconscious Blocks: Inherited stories of shame, sexual repression, or fear of judgment can lead to an inability to connect fully with one's body and sexual experiences. Addressing these imprints through womb healing can help women release these blocks, allowing for deeper connection and pleasure.

7. Microbial Infections and Vaginal Health

Frequent microbial infections in the vagina can also be viewed as a manifestation of energetic and emotional imbalance. The vaginal microbiome is highly sensitive to stress, hormonal fluctuations, and emotional states. Chronic stress or unresolved trauma can weaken the immune response and disrupt the natural balance of beneficial bacteria, leading to infections.

Emotional and Spiritual Aspects:

Infections can sometimes symbolize an energetic boundary breach or unresolved emotions manifesting physically. If a woman feels violated, unheard, or emotionally burdened, the body may respond through physical imbalance in its most vulnerable areas.

Inherited Trauma and Shame:

Generational shame or guilt surrounding sexuality and womanhood can create a "hostile" internal environment where infections thrive, reflecting a need for cleansing and reconnection with one's body.

8. Uterine, Ovarian, and Cervical Cancer

Medical Aspect: These cancers involve complex genetic, environmental, and lifestyle factors.

Cancers of the reproductive organs are complex and multifactorial, often involving genetic, environmental, and lifestyle factors. However, from a holistic and energetic perspective, these cancers can be seen as the body signaling deep-seated, unresolved trauma, anger, or grief that has festered over time.

Suppressed Emotions: Suppression of creativity, unresolved anger, grief, or unprocessed emotions can create an environment of energetic stagnation. This stagnation may manifest as cellular imbalance, contributing to the development of tumors and cancerous growths.

Generational Imprints and Ancestral Pain: Cancer in the womb, ovaries, or cervix may reflect the manifestation of deeply held generational pain, shame, or betrayal. It can be a physical manifestation of centuries of oppression, suppression of the feminine voice, or unhealed traumas passed down through family lines.

Cancerous growth can be interpreted as the body's attempt to cope with profound disruptions in its natural rhythm. Chronic stress, hormonal imbalances, lack of self-expression, and the denial of one's true desires and emotions all contribute to this loss of rhythm, creating an environment where disease can take root.

The Common Thread: Loss of Natural Rhythm

All these conditions—whether vaginal dryness, difficulty with orgasm, microbial infections, or reproductive cancers—highlight a loss of the body's natural rhythm and balance. When a woman's life becomes dominated by stress, societal pressures, unprocessed emotions, and inherited traumas, her body responds by manifesting imbalance in the organs most closely tied to her feminine energy. The womb and reproductive organs, as centers of creation and life, often bear the brunt of these imbalances.

Reconnecting to Natural Rhythms:

Healing involves more than addressing physical symptoms; it requires reconnecting with one's natural cycles, rhythms, and the feminine essence. Practices such as womb meditation, emotional release techniques, mindfulness, and honoring one's cycles can help restore balance and invite healing.

Emotional Release and Healing Trauma:
By addressing the root causes of energetic, emotional, and ancestral imbalances, women can begin to restore their natural flow and rhythm. This may involve releasing inherited trauma, confronting suppressed emotions, and creating a supportive environment for true healing. As we view these conditions through the lens of energetic and ancestral imprints helps us understand that physical symptoms often have deeper roots in our emotional, generational, and energetic histories. When the natural rhythm of the body is disrupted—by stress, trauma, societal pressures, or inherited beliefs—the body

responds by manifesting imbalance. Healing involves reconnecting with the feminine essence, addressing both inherited and personal trauma, and restoring harmony within the body, mind, and spirit. This approach can empower women to reclaim their health, vitality, and authentic selves.

Case Studies: The Connection Between Unresolved Emotional Pain and Physical Health

The following case studies demonstrate the connection between unresolved emotional pain and physical symptoms in the womb, highlighting how addressing these emotional and generational patterns can contribute to healing.

Case Study 1: Healing Fibroids Through Emotional Release

Maria, came to me struggling with painful fibroids that impacted her daily life. Through our sessions, she revealed a history of suppressing her emotions, particularly anger and frustration about unmet needs in her family. Maria felt she had to keep everyone happy, suppressing her voice and ignoring her own desires. She realized that her fibroids symbolized this suppression and her repressed need to express herself.

Together, we worked on releasing her suppressed emotions through journaling, guided visualizations, and somatic exercises that helped her reconnect with her body. Maria began expressing herself freely and made choices aligned with her true desires. Over time, her fibroid symptoms decreased, and she reported feeling physically lighter and emotionally liberated.

Case Study 2: Addressing PCOS and Embracing Feminine Energy

Sophia, a client diagnosed with PCOS, came to recognize her disconnection from femininity as a root issue. She had always felt that embracing feminine qualities was a sign of weakness and had overcompensated by embodying traits society deemed strong and masculine. This inner conflict manifested in hormonal imbalances, irregular periods, and low self-worth.

In her healing journey, we focused on reclaiming her feminine essence, using practices like womb meditation, energy work, and affirmations to encourage acceptance of her femininity. As she began to embrace this energy, her cycle gradually normalized, and her hormonal levels balanced. Sophia reported feeling a newfound sense of self-worth and began to honor her feminine traits as a source of strength.

Case Study 3: Releasing Generational Trauma to Support Fertility

Priya, struggled with unexplained infertility despite being physically healthy. Through deep trance work and inner child healing, she discovered that her maternal lineage carried unresolved grief from losing children and experiencing abandonment. Priya realized she had subconsciously inherited these fears, creating an inner block against becoming a mother.

Using ancestral healing techniques, Priya connected with her lineage, honoring their pain and consciously choosing to release it. She performed regular womb-cleansing rituals and set intentions to create a new path free from inherited fears. Within a year, Priya conceived naturally, feeling that the healing work had lifted the emotional barrier that had prevented her from embracing motherhood fully.

Case Study 4: Menstrual Pain and Releasing Shame

Ayesha experienced severe menstrual pain and irregular cycles, often accompanied by debilitating cramps. In our sessions, she revealed a deep-rooted sense of shame and discomfort around menstruation due to negative societal beliefs she had absorbed from her upbringing. We worked on reframing her relationship with her cycle through rituals, self-acceptance practices, and releasing inherited shame around menstruation. As she cultivated a healthier connection with her body, her menstrual cycles stabilized, and her pain significantly lessened.

Case Study 5: Restoring Feminine Flow and Addressing Vaginal Dryness

Healing vaginal dryness involves more than addressing the physical symptoms. It requires exploring and releasing the emotional, psychological, and energetic blocks that contribute to resistance to sexual pleasure.

When Elena faced chronic vaginal dryness, which impacted her intimacy and overall well-being, we began to identify and release feelings of shame or guilt associated with sexuality. Upon exploring the issue, we hit a forgotten memory of sexual abuse which led to a disconnection from her feminine essence and sensuality. By counseling, trauma-informed therapy, and holistic practices that focus on releasing stored emotions, Elena was able to feel safe and reconnect with her sexuality.

Case Study 6: Difficulty Achieving Orgasm and Releasing Shame

When Meera confided that she struggled with achieving orgasm only during intercourse, I knew there was a deeper puzzle that needed unraveling. Through our work together, it became clear that she had inherited beliefs about sexual repression from her mother, who, in turn, had absorbed a patriarchal notion that sexual pleasure was reserved solely for men. This generational belief system had unconsciously shaped Meera's perception of her own sexuality, creating barriers to fully experiencing intimacy and pleasure. Meera was determined to break this cycle. As she prepared to start a family, she recognized that healing these deeply rooted beliefs was not only essential for herself but also for future generations. Her commitment to change was profound. Together, we worked to identify and address her subconscious fears, reframing inherited narratives around pleasure, sexuality, and worthiness. Through guided bodywork, affirmations, and gentle exploration of her emotional landscape, Meera began to shed the layers of shame and repression that had held her back.

Case Study 7: Chronic Microbial Infections and Emotional Boundaries

Carla experienced frequent microbial infections that significantly disrupted her life. Upon exploration, we discovered that she harbored unacknowledged fears around becoming a mother, stemming from the pressures and sacrifices she witnessed in her own upbringing. Additionally, Carla often felt that her boundaries were violated in relationships and struggled with asserting her own needs.

Our work focused on identifying and releasing these underlying beliefs and fears, using visualization techniques, emotional release practices, and affirmations to strengthen her boundaries and reconnect her with her authentic desires. As Carla began to assert herself and redefine her vision of motherhood, she noticed significant improvements in her vaginal health. By addressing the root causes of her subconscious resistance, Carla was able to restore balance to her body and create an environment that naturally repelled harmful bacteria, reflecting her newfound emotional clarity and empowerment.

Case Study 8: Releasing Anger and Healing Cancerous Growths

Anita was diagnosed with cervical cancer and sought support for emotional healing alongside medical treatment. Through her journey, she uncovered deeply held anger and grief tied to past relationships and generational pain. By using emotional release techniques, forgiveness practices, and working through ancestral healing, she felt a profound emotional shift. Anita reported a greater sense of peace and purpose, and her healing journey became an integrated part of her cancer treatment process.

Summary: Chapter 3

Recognizing the physical manifestations of womb imbalances is essential in understanding how deeply emotions, trauma, and generational patterns influence our health. While these conditions often have medical explanations, looking beneath the surface reveals emotional and spiritual roots that can provide insights and pathways to healing. Through womb healing practices that integrate emotional release, subconscious reprogramming, and ancestral healing, women can begin to address the underlying causes of these physical imbalances.

Each woman's journey is unique, but the common thread is the powerful interplay between the body, emotions, and ancestral history. Womb healing offers a path to reconnect with these layers, releasing what no longer serves and allowing physical health and emotional balance to emerge naturally.

Chapter 4: Releasing Emotional Trauma Stored in the Womb

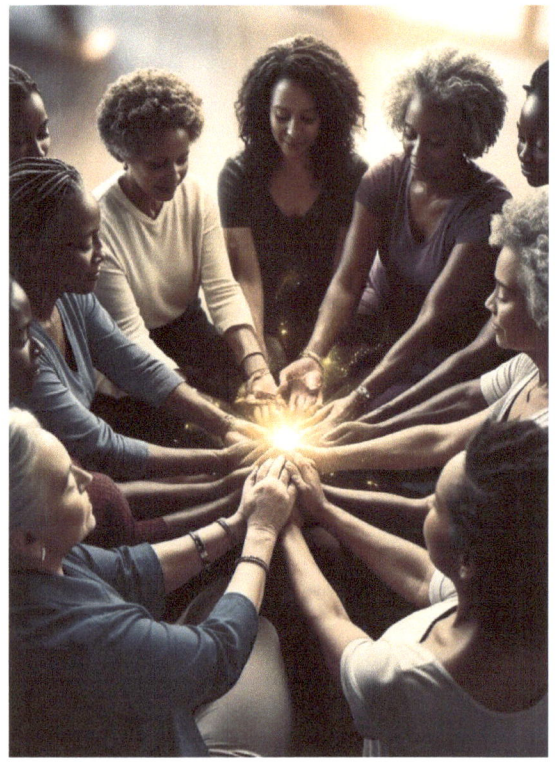

The womb, as a sacred center of feminine energy, carries not only the potential for physical creation but also the emotional imprints of life experiences. Traumas, particularly those involving shame, grief, and feelings of inadequacy, tend to settle deep within the womb, creating blockages that impact physical, emotional, and spiritual health. Understanding how these emotional traumas are stored and learning to release them can lead to profound healing and reconnection with the self and the restoration of feminine power.

Emotional Trauma in the Body and the Womb

Emotional trauma leaves its imprint not only on the mind but also on the body, particularly in areas linked to our emotions and reproductive systems. For women, the womb becomes a repository for unprocessed emotions, often manifesting as pain, tension, or imbalance. Feelings of inadequacy, shame, and grief—whether arising from personal experiences or passed down through generations—tend to accumulate in this space, subtly shaping beliefs, behaviors, and overall health.

Inadequacy: Societal and relational pressures frequently create a sense of "not enough" within women. Unrealistic beauty standards, the burden of fulfilling multiple roles, or experiences of rejection contribute to this pervasive feeling, which settles into the body, influencing self-worth and self-image.

Shame: Criticism, judgment, and trauma related to intimacy and sexuality can generate deep-rooted shame. This shame often resides in the womb, suppressing creativity and connection to one's feminine essence.

Grief: The loss of loved ones, unfulfilled desires for motherhood, or inherited generational pain can manifest as grief stored in the womb. This grief may linger, impacting physical health and emotional well-being.

Research shows that unexpressed or unprocessed emotions are stored in the body (Van der Kolk, *The Body Keeps the Score*). The womb, as a highly sensitive center, is particularly vulnerable to these imprints. When left unaddressed, they can manifest as chronic pelvic pain, menstrual irregularities, or reproductive health conditions. Recognizing and releasing these emotional traumas paves the way for healing on multiple levels, reestablishing a connection to power, creativity, and self-worth.

Practices for Emotional Release

Releasing emotional trauma stored in the womb requires practices that access the subconscious, help us process unexpressed emotions, and create a safe space for healing. Here are three effective practices:

journaling, inner child healing, and mindfulness exercises.

1. Journaling for Emotional Release

Journaling is a powerful tool for uncovering and releasing hidden emotions. Through writing, we can express thoughts and feelings we may otherwise repress, allowing us to confront and understand our emotional wounds.

➢ Journaling Prompts:

"What experiences in my life have made me feel inadequate? How did I internalize those feelings?"

"Are there any memories related to shame or judgment that I feel in my womb? How can I show myself compassion for those experiences?"

"What aspects of my life have brought grief to my womb space? How can I allow myself to grieve openly?"

➢ Spend time reflecting on each question.

Write freely without judgment, letting emotions surface as you go. The goal is not to analyze but to release—this is a space to honor your feelings without censoring them.

Inner Child Healing

Many of our emotional wounds stem from childhood experiences and subconscious beliefs formed early in life. Inner child healing involves connecting with our younger selves, offering them understanding and compassion, and releasing the emotional burdens they carry.

Inner Child Exercise:

Close your eyes, take a few deep breaths, and picture yourself as a child. See this child within a safe, comforting space. Imagine speaking with this younger self, asking them what they need to feel safe and loved. Allow any emotions to arise, acknowledging them with compassion. Visualize embracing this child, reassuring them that they are worthy, loved, and enough just as they are. Tell them that they no longer need to carry the burden of shame or inadequacy.

This exercise can be done regularly to help release subconscious emotions that may be contributing to emotional trauma in the womb.

Mindfulness and Body Awareness

Mindfulness exercises help bring awareness to sensations in the body, allowing you to observe and release tension, discomfort, or emotions stored in the womb.

Mindfulness Exercise:

Sit or lie comfortably and bring your awareness to your breath, feeling it move through your body.

Slowly direct your attention to your womb, noticing any sensations or emotions that arise.

If you sense tightness, pain, or discomfort, breathe into that area. With each exhale, visualize releasing any tension or emotion held there.

Gently remind yourself that it is safe to let go. Imagine a warm light filling the womb, bringing comfort, healing, and peace.

Guided Meditation for Emotional Release

This meditation is designed to facilitate emotional release from the womb, focusing on forgiveness, self-compassion, and acceptance. Find a quiet place where you won't be disturbed, sit or lie down comfortably, and close your eyes.

Guided Meditation Steps

➢ Ground and Center:

Begin by taking several deep breaths, inhaling slowly through your nose and exhaling gently through your mouth.
With each breath, feel yourself becoming more relaxed and centered. Picture roots growing from your body into the earth, grounding you.

➢ Connect with the Womb Space:

Gently bring your awareness to your womb. Picture it as a warm, glowing space within your lower abdomen.
Visualize a soft, nurturing light within the womb. This light is warm and comforting, gently illuminating the area.

➢ Identify Emotions to Release:

Silently ask your womb if it holds any emotions that are ready to be released. Trust whatever arises, whether it's a specific feeling, memory, or sensation.

Acknowledge any emotions that come up, such as inadequacy, shame, or grief, without judgment. Imagine these emotions as dark clouds or shapes within the light of your womb.

➢ Focus on Forgiveness:

As you breathe, focus on forgiveness—not just for others, but for yourself. Silently say to yourself, *"I forgive myself for carrying these burdens."*
Picture the dark clouds or shapes gradually dissolving into the warm light, transformed by forgiveness and understanding.

➢ Invite Self-Compassion:

Now, direct feelings of compassion toward your womb. Silently say, *"I show myself compassion for every wound and every experience stored here."*

Imagine the light within your womb growing warmer and brighter, filling every corner with compassion and gentleness.

➢ Embrace Acceptance:

With each inhale, breathe in acceptance for yourself and your journey. Silently affirm,

"I accept myself as I am, and I release what no longer serves me."

Picture any remaining emotions flowing out of your womb, leaving a sense of peace, openness, and lightness in their place.

➢ Close with Gratitude:

Bring your attention back to your breath, feeling the grounding energy from the earth supporting you.

Place your hands over your womb and take a moment to express gratitude for this sacred space within you. Silently say,

"Thank you, my womb, for holding my emotions and guiding my healing."

➢ Return to the Present:

Gently wiggle your fingers and toes, gradually bringing your awareness back to the room. When you're ready, open your eyes, feeling grounded and at peace.

Summary: Chapter 4

Releasing emotional trauma stored in the womb is a powerful step toward reclaiming inner strength and self-worth. Emotions such as inadequacy, shame, and grief need not remain buried within; they can be acknowledged, honored, and gently released. Through practices like journaling, inner child healing, mindfulness, and guided meditation, we create a nurturing environment for deep emotional healing. Womb healing transforms a place of pain into a source of empowerment, creativity, and peace, reconnecting us with our true selves and allowing us to embrace life with renewed freedom, love, and self-compassion. Womb healing allows us to reconnect with our deepest selves, turning a place of pain into a source of empowerment and peace. Each practice serves as a bridge to self-compassion, forgiveness, and acceptance, allowing us to let go of past burdens and embrace a life of emotional freedom, creativity, **and self-love.**

Chapter 5: Reclaiming Your Feminine Power Through Subconscious Reprogramming

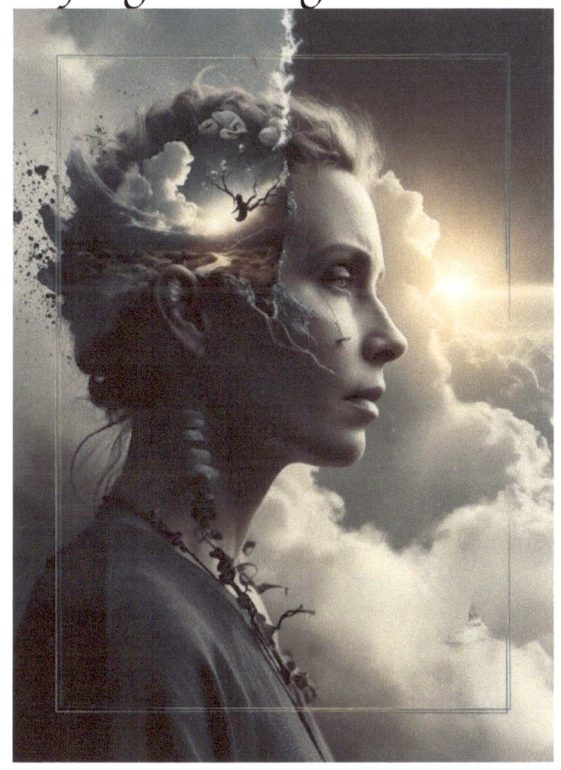

Reclaiming feminine power often requires a shift at the deepest levels of the subconscious mind, where our beliefs about worth, identity, and self-expression are stored. For centuries, women have been conditioned by societal narratives that restrict the ways they can express their power, beauty, and wisdom. These messages often form limiting beliefs, keeping women from fully embodying their potential. Through subconscious reprogramming, we can begin dismantling these inherited and internalized beliefs, opening the path to self-acceptance, empowerment, and true connection with feminine energy.

Subconscious Programming Techniques for Reclaiming Power

The subconscious mind operates beneath our awareness, yet it shapes much of our perception, behavior, and self-identity. We absorb messages from early life experiences, cultural norms, family dynamics, and past traumas that unconsciously influence our sense of worth and power. Subconscious programming techniques are designed to help bring these beliefs to light and replace them with ones that reflect our true value and potential. Some key methods for subconscious reprogramming include:

1. **Affirmations**: Repeating positive statements designed to override limiting beliefs and rewire the subconscious mind.

2. **Visualization**: Engaging the imagination to create empowering images and scenarios that shift perceptions and build confidence.

3. **Hypnotherapy**: Using a deeply relaxed, trance-like state to access and alter subconscious beliefs directly.

4. **Meditative Self-Inquiry**: Reflecting on deeply held beliefs through meditation to uncover and challenge unhelpful assumptions.

The goal of these techniques is to address limiting beliefs about self-worth, identity, and feminine power. For example, a woman who believes she is "not enough" may constantly doubt her abilities and avoid expressing her needs. Through subconscious reprogramming, she can replace this belief with one of inherent worth, empowering her to act with confidence.

Dismantling Internalized Societal Messages

For generations, women have been subjected to societal narratives that dictate how they should look, behave, and think. These narratives often emphasize self-sacrifice, silence, and compliance, limiting women's expressions of independence and power. Many women carry subconscious messages such as "I am only valued if I am serving others," "I should not speak up," or "I must be perfect to be loved." These beliefs can limit their potential and restrict their authenticity.

To dismantle these internalized messages, we must first identify them. One effective technique is to practice **Thought Awareness Journaling**.

This involves:

1. **Document Automatic Thoughts**: Over a week, keep a journal of recurring thoughts, particularly those that evoke self-doubt, shame, or fear.

2. **Identify Patterns**: Identify any patterns or themes. Are there thoughts that relate to not being enough, fearing judgment, or questioning one's power?

3. **Challenge and Reframe Beliefs**: Ask yourself, "Where did I learn this?" or "Is this belief truly mine, or was it imposed by society?" Recognize that many of these beliefs are inherited rather than authentic. Once you've identified these internalized messages, **Affirmation Reframing** can be an effective tool for subconscious reprogramming:

4. **Create Empowering Affirmations**: For each limiting belief, create an affirmation that directly counters it. For instance, replace "I am only valued if I am serving others" with "I am valuable simply as I am, and my needs are important."

5. **Daily Repetition**: Repeat these affirmations each morning and evening, ideally in front of a mirror to reinforce self-acceptance.

Over time, these affirmations recondition the mind to accept new, empowering beliefs. Studies on neural plasticity have shown that consistent repetition can reshape the brain's pathways, allowing these new beliefs to become second nature (Doidge, *The Brain That Changes Itself*).

Cultivating Empowering Beliefs About Womanhood, Motherhood, and Self-Worth

Reclaiming feminine power involves creating new beliefs about what it means to be a woman, especially around aspects like womanhood, motherhood, and self-worth. These are often areas most heavily influenced by societal expectations, leaving women with distorted views of their value and purpose. By intentionally cultivating empowering beliefs, we realign with our true essence and inner wisdom.

Here are exercises designed to help develop and embody these beliefs:

Embracing Womanhood:

1. *Exercise*: **Goddess Visualization**

Sit in a comfortable position and close your eyes. Visualize a powerful, radiant goddess who embodies everything you believe a strong, empowered woman should be.

Picture her grace, wisdom, compassion, and strength.

Imagine her approaching you and placing her hands over your womb, filling you with the qualities she embodies.

Affirm silently, "I am a woman of power, beauty, and grace. I embrace my feminine essence in all its forms."

This practice allows you to embody qualities you admire, grounding these traits within yourself.

Redefining Motherhood:

Exercise: **Mother Archetype Reflection**

Reflect on the beliefs you hold about motherhood, whether or not you are a mother. Write down any limiting messages, such as "A good mother sacrifices herself" or "My worth is tied to my children's success."

For each message, create an empowering belief, such as "Motherhood is a part of me, not my whole identity" or "I nurture myself as I nurture others."

Use these beliefs to develop new affirmations that honor a balanced, empowered view of motherhood.

Affirming Self-Worth:

Exercise: **Self-Worth Mirror Work**

Stand in front of a mirror, look into your own eyes, and state aloud, "I am worthy of love, respect, and success. My worth is intrinsic and independent of others' opinions."

Repeat this daily, especially when self-doubt arises. Visualize each word settling into your subconscious, helping to dismantle old beliefs of inadequacy. This exercise helps strengthen self-worth by connecting with oneself directly, allowing these affirmations to bypass self-doubt and root deeply in the subconscious.

Subconscious Reprogramming Meditation for Feminine Power

This meditation guides you to connect with your subconscious and release limiting beliefs around feminine power, replacing them with affirmations of worth and strength.

Settle and Ground: Find a comfortable place to sit. Close your eyes, take several deep breaths, and imagine roots extending from your body into the earth, grounding you.

Visualize Your Womb as a Place of Power: Imagine a warm, golden light in your womb area. This is your center of creation and strength. Feel it growing, radiating power and confidence through your body.

Identify Limiting Beliefs: Bring to mind any beliefs about yourself as a woman that feel limiting or self-defeating. Visualize each belief as a dark mist around your womb, holding the energy of old narratives.

Release and Transform: With each exhale, visualize this mist dissolving, dissipating into the light of your womb. Feel the beliefs losing their hold, replaced by feelings of freedom and empowerment.

Affirm Your Worth and Power: Silently repeat, "I am powerful. I am worthy. I embody the full essence of womanhood." Feel each word resonate deeply within your subconscious.

Anchor Your New Beliefs: Imagine the light in your womb expanding to fill your entire body, creating a radiant aura around you. With each breath, this new, empowered energy solidifies in your being.

Summary: Chapter 5

Subconscious reprogramming is a journey of returning to the truth of who we are, free from inherited limitations and societal conditioning. By embracing techniques such as affirmations, visualization, and mirror work, we replace old beliefs with new narratives of empowerment, redefining womanhood, motherhood, and self-worth in ways that honor our full potential.

As you continue to use these practices, remember that reprogramming the subconscious is a gradual process. Be patient with yourself, celebrate each small shift, and recognize the strength that emerges from within as you reclaim your feminine power. This journey allows you not only to heal but also to thrive, bringing forth the innate wisdom and creativity that reside in every woman.

Chapter 6: Healing Generational Inadequacies and Breaking Cycles

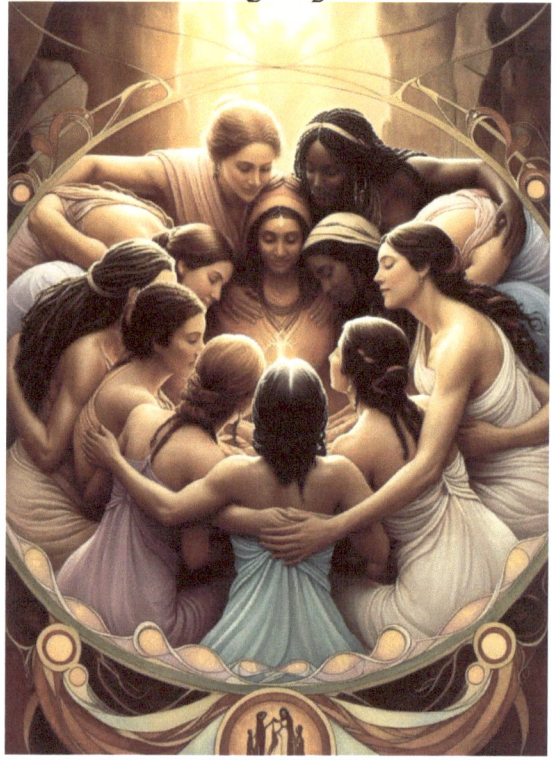

Our bodies and minds carry not only our own stories but also those of our ancestors. Generational patterns of inadequacy, neglect, and suppression are passed down through families, imprinted within us as unconscious beliefs, emotional responses, and even physical conditions. In order to fully reclaim our personal worth, we must first acknowledge and heal these inherited wounds. This chapter provides methods to identify generational patterns, offers a guided trance meditation to connect with and release ancestral pain, and encourages a transformation of inherited experiences into sources of personal and collective strength.

Identifying Generational Patterns of Inadequacy, Neglect, or Suppression

The first step in healing generational inadequacies is recognizing these patterns within ourselves. Generational patterns often manifest as recurring thoughts, behaviors, or emotional responses that feel instinctual, yet misaligned with who we aspire to be. These inherited beliefs and reactions may come from experiences of inadequacy, neglect, or suppression in our ancestral line. Identifying and acknowledging these patterns is key to breaking the cycle. Here are some ways to identify generational patterns in your life:

Reflect on Family Narratives:

Take time to reflect on the messages you grew up hearing about worth, success, and personal identity. Common themes like "Our family is not meant for greatness," or "We are always struggling," may be indications of deeply rooted beliefs carried from previous generations. Notice any recurring phrases or sentiments that reflect limiting beliefs or feelings of inadequacy.

Observe Emotional Triggers and Patterns:

Pay attention to recurring emotional patterns, especially feelings of inadequacy, fear of failure, or self-doubt. These emotions may feel instinctual, arising even in situations where they are not rational. If you experience disproportionate reactions to certain situations, consider whether these reactions may stem from generational trauma or beliefs rather than your own experiences. Identifying these patterns can help distinguish between what is truly yours and what has been passed down.

Family History of Suppression or Trauma:

Examine any known experiences of hardship, discrimination, or trauma within your family history. Events such as war, economic hardship, or systemic oppression often leave deep emotional imprints that are carried forward by descendants. Speak with family members to uncover significant experiences that may have contributed to generational patterns of suppression, fear, or inadequacy. Ask family members about significant events in your family's past, particularly those related to suppression or adversity.

Body-Centered Awareness:

Sometimes, generational patterns manifest as physical sensations, such as tension, heaviness, or discomfort in certain parts of the body—especially in the womb or lower abdomen, where emotions are stored. Use body-centered mindfulness to notice where you may be holding tension or heaviness, as these sensations can point to unprocessed generational trauma.

Once you have identified these patterns, write them down. Recognizing them is the first step toward releasing them and creating space for new beliefs and healthier responses.

A Deep Trance Meditation to Connect with Ancestral Energies and Release Inherited Feelings of Inadequacy

This guided trance meditation is designed to help you connect with your ancestral lineage, recognize inherited patterns of inadequacy, and release them from your energetic and emotional space.

Preparation:

➢ Find a quiet, comfortable place where you won't be disturbed. Sit or lie down in a position that allows you to relax deeply.

➢ Set an intention, such as *"I release all inherited feelings of inadequacy and reclaim my worth and strength."*

Meditation Steps:

Entering a Trance State:

Close your eyes and take a few deep breaths, inhaling through your nose and exhaling slowly through your mouth. Begin counting down from ten to one, allowing each number to relax you further, bringing you into a deep, peaceful state.

Imagine yourself descending a staircase, going deeper with each step, feeling safe and calm.

Creating a Sacred Ancestral Space:
Visualize yourself in a beautiful, tranquil place—a sacred space that feels comforting and secure. This could be a meadow, a quiet forest, or any place that brings you peace.

Imagine that before you stands a pathway surrounded by gentle light, leading you to your ancestral lineage.

Inviting Your Ancestors to Appear:
Silently invite your ancestors to join you, asking them to reveal themselves in this sacred space. Allow yourself to feel their presence. You may see or sense them standing before you in a line, stretching far into the distance.

With a compassionate heart, acknowledge their presence and the lives they led.

Observing Generational Patterns:

In your mind, ask them to reveal any feelings of inadequacy, neglect, or suppression that have been passed down through your lineage. Notice if any patterns or emotions come forward. These may appear as shadows, images, words, or simply feelings.

Take your time to sense any pain, sadness, or limitation they may have carried. Allow yourself to honor their experiences, knowing they faced these challenges with strength and resilience.

Offering Healing and Releasing Inadequacies:

Visualize a warm, golden light filling your heart, representing love, compassion, and healing. Allow this light to expand and radiate out toward your ancestors, sending them the energy of acceptance, peace, and release.

Imagine the light flowing through them, dissolving any feelings of inadequacy, neglect, or suppression they carried. As the light fills each ancestor, see them becoming lighter, freer, and more at peace.

Reclaiming Your Own Worth and Strength:

Now, bring your focus back to yourself. Imagine the golden light flowing back to you, filling your womb or lower abdomen with warmth and strength. Allow this light to dissolve any feelings of inadequacy that have been passed down, reclaiming your inherent worth and strength.

Silently affirm, "I release all inherited inadequacies and stand strong in my own worth. I am whole, complete, and empowered."

Expressing Gratitude and Closing the Space:

Thank your ancestors for sharing their stories and allowing healing to take place. Visualize them peacefully fading back into the light, with the sense that they are now free, their love and blessings remaining with you.

Slowly bring your awareness back to your breath and the present moment. Take a few deep breaths, feeling grounded, empowered, and connected to a lineage of strength.

Returning to Awareness:

Gently open your eyes when you feel ready. Take a few minutes to write down any insights or feelings that arose during the meditation.

Summary: Chapter 6

As you begin to recognize and heal generational patterns, it's essential to honor your lineage, understanding that their experiences have contributed to the person you are today. The pain they endured, the challenges they faced, and the strength they demonstrated all play a part in shaping your identity. When you release inherited inadequacies, you are not rejecting your lineage but rather healing and honoring it in a new way.

Consider incorporating practices that honor your ancestors as part of your ongoing healing journey. This could be as simple as lighting a candle in their memory, speaking words of gratitude, or journaling about the strength and resilience they exhibited. By acknowledging both their struggles and their triumphs, you transform inherited pain into a source of strength and resilience within yourself.

Remember, healing generational trauma is not a rejection of the past but an evolution of it. As you release patterns of inadequacy, you make space for empowerment, strength, and worth, passing these gifts onto future generations. Embracing this journey creates a ripple effect, healing not only your life but also the collective feminine energy that flows through all of us.

Chapter 7: Integrating Womb Healing with Energy Practices

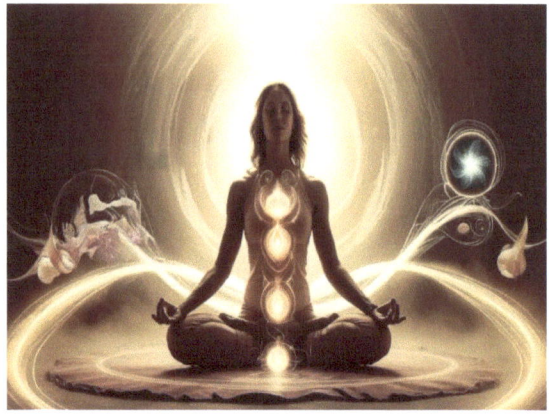

Energy-based practices are profound tools for womb healing, helping to clear, balance, and recharge the womb space. By engaging techniques like reiki, chakra balancing, and breathwork, we can release stagnant energy, invite deep healing, and sustain a vibrant connection to our creative center. These practices not only support physical and emotional wellness but also cultivate a powerful connection to our feminine essence. This chapter explores these techniques in depth, along with guided visualization exercises, empowering readers to develop rituals that honor and nurture their womb space.

Energy-Based Practices for Womb Healing

Energy practices can be powerful allies in womb healing, as they work with the subtle body to release deep-seated emotional blocks, balance our energy centers, and connect us to a state of inner peace and vitality. Here, we'll cover three practices that are especially effective for supporting womb health and well-being.

1. Reiki for Womb Healing

Reiki, a form of energy healing that originated in Japan, involves channeling healing energy to cleanse and balance the body's energetic fields. By placing hands over the womb area and allowing the reiki energy to flow, one can release negative emotions, trauma, and stagnant energy held within the womb.

How to Perform Reiki on the Womb:

Find a Quiet Space: Sit or lie down comfortably, closing your eyes and setting an intention for womb healing.

Warm Your Hands: Rub your palms together to activate energy in your hands.

Place Your Hands on Your Lower Abdomen: Gently place your hands over your womb area, just below your navel.

Visualize Light Energy: Imagine a warm, golden light flowing from your hands into your womb, filling it with healing energy.

Feel the Flow: As the energy flows, visualize it releasing any dark or heavy energy from your womb. Imagine these energies dissolving into the light.

Close with Gratitude: After a few minutes, remove your hands, and express gratitude for the healing received. This practice can be done for 5-10 minutes daily or whenever you feel the need for emotional release.

2. Chakra Balancing for the Sacral and Root Chakras

The sacral and root chakras are directly linked to womb health. The sacral chakra, located just below the navel, governs creativity, sexuality, and emotional expression. The root chakra, located at the base of the spine, is our foundation for safety and security. Keeping these two chakras balanced supports a healthy flow of energy to the womb, providing emotional and physical stability.

Sacral Chakra Balancing:

Visualization: Sit comfortably and close your eyes. Visualize a warm orange light glowing in your lower abdomen. Imagine this orange light expanding, filling your womb and lower belly with vibrant energy.

Affirmations: Silently repeat affirmations such as "I am creative," "I am emotionally balanced," and "I embrace my feminine power."

Breathing: Take deep breaths, feeling the orange light strengthening with each inhale. As you exhale, release any emotional tension.

Root Chakra Balancing:

Visualization: Focus on the base of your spine. Imagine a deep red light here, representing stability and groundedness. Visualize this red light anchoring you to the earth, providing support and safety.

Affirmations: Repeat affirmations like "I am safe," "I am grounded," and "I trust the journey of life."

Breathing: As you breathe deeply, feel the red light strengthening your connection to the earth, grounding and stabilizing your energy.

Together, these visualizations help create a balanced flow between the sacral and root chakras, supporting both the emotional and physical aspects of womb health.

3. Breathwork for Clearing and Energizing the Womb

Breathwork is a powerful practice for releasing stored emotions and revitalizing the energy of the womb. It involves using focused breath to move energy, bringing clarity, calm, and healing.

Womb Breathwork:

Sit Comfortably: Place your hands on your lower abdomen and close your eyes.

Deep Belly Breaths: Inhale deeply through your nose, expanding your belly and filling your womb space with oxygen and energy.

Exhale Slowly: Release the breath slowly through your mouth, imagining any stress or negative emotions leaving your body.

Visualize Cleansing: With each inhale, imagine a soft, white light entering your womb, purifying and energizing it. With each exhale, visualize any dark, heavy energy being released.

Repeat: Continue this breathwork for 5-10 minutes, focusing on filling your womb with healing light and releasing any stored tension.

Guided Womb Visualization and Energy Cleansing

This visualization practice is designed to help you connect deeply with your womb, clearing away any stagnant energy and inviting healing light into this sacred space.

Create a Calm Environment: Find a quiet space and sit or lie down comfortably.

Close your eyes and take a few deep breaths, allowing yourself to relax.

Visualize Your Womb Space: Bring your awareness to your womb, just below the navel. Imagine this area as a warm, soft space, like a small room within you.

Observe the Energy: Gently observe the energy in this space. You may notice colors, sensations, or symbols representing stored emotions, memories, or beliefs. Trust whatever appears, without judgment.

Cleansing Light: Imagine a golden or white light entering your womb space. This light gently clears away any dark or heavy energies, dissolving them into the light. Visualize the energy within your womb becoming clearer, brighter, and lighter.

Fill with Positive Energy: Once the cleansing feels complete, visualize your womb filling with warm, vibrant energy. Imagine this energy radiating throughout your body, bringing a sense of peace, wholeness, and strength.

Close the Visualization: When you feel ready, slowly bring your awareness back to the present. Place your hands over your womb and express gratitude for the healing and connection you've experienced.

Creating a Daily Ritual for Honoring the Womb

A daily ritual is a powerful way to maintain an ongoing connection with your womb, fostering its energetic balance and honoring it as a sacred space within you.

Daily Womb Honoring Ritual:

1. Morning Connection:

Place Your Hands on Your Womb: Upon waking, place your hands on your lower abdomen and take a few deep breaths, feeling the rise and fall of your womb with each breath.

Set an Intention: Set an intention for the day, such as "I honor my feminine power" or "I embrace my creativity and intuition."

Gratitude: Spend a moment in gratitude for your body and your womb, acknowledging its power and presence.

2. Midday Pause:

Grounding Breath: Take a short pause midday to ground yourself. Place your hands on your womb and take a few deep breaths, letting go of any stress or tension.

Affirmation: Repeat an affirmation, like "I am centered" or "I am balanced and peaceful."

3. Evening Reflection:

Womb Cleansing: Before bed, visualize a gentle white light flowing into your womb, cleansing away any stress, worry, or tension accumulated throughout the day.

Express Gratitude: Take a moment to thank your womb for the wisdom, strength, and creativity it holds, setting the intention to continue nurturing and honoring this sacred space.

By creating a daily ritual, you foster an ongoing relationship with your womb, deepening your connection to your feminine essence and maintaining its energetic balance. This practice not only supports your emotional and physical health but also helps you stay in tune with your inner wisdom and creativity.

These practices—when integrated into your life—can transform how you experience yourself and the world, creating a strong, balanced, and vibrant connection with the sacred womb.

Summary of Chapter 7:

Chapter 7 highlights the transformative power of energy-based practices in womb healing, offering tools to clear, balance, and recharge the womb space. These practices not only release deep-seated emotional blocks but also nurture a vibrant connection to one's feminine essence. Key techniques explored include:

Reiki for Womb Healing
Chakra Balancing for Sacral and Root Chakras
Breathwork for Energizing the Womb
Guided Visualization for Womb Cleansing
Daily Womb Honoring Rituals

Chapter 8: Reconnecting with Creative and Sexual Energy

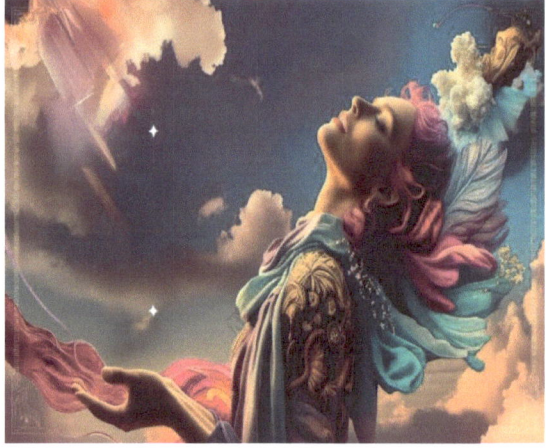

The journey of womb healing brings us back to a profound connection with our creative and sexual energy, energies that are intimately linked. The womb is not only a physical organ but also an energetic center where life, creativity, and sensuality merge. Reconnecting with this sacred space allows us to embrace our full potential, honoring our sensuality, creativity, and power as expressions of who we truly are.

The Connection Between the Womb and Creative, Sensual Energy

The womb is the source of feminine energy, where creativity and sensuality arise from the same deep well. Just as the womb nurtures new life, it is also a wellspring for creative ideas, artistic expression, and the pleasure of living fully. Our creative impulses and our capacity for sensuality stem from this center, both requiring openness, receptivity, and the courage to feel deeply.

When we are connected to our wombs, we are connected to the essence of creation itself. This is why creative energy is so often described as a "birthing" process, whether it involves the creation of art, new ideas, or even a sense of self. Creativity and sensuality are closely intertwined, as both require us to trust our inner impulses and surrender to flow. Sensuality, in this context, is not limited to sexuality but encompasses all our senses—the joy of tasting, seeing, hearing, touching, and experiencing life.

Yet for many women, this connection becomes blocked by past experiences of shame, guilt, or societal conditioning. Cultural messages have often diminished or stigmatized feminine sexuality and creativity, leading many women to feel disconnected from their own bodies and desires. Reclaiming our creative and sexual energy is therefore an act of empowerment, a way to reconnect with the fullness of our being and to live from a place of authenticity and joy.

Consider Your Womb and Body as Sacred

In this journey of reconnecting with your creative and sexual energy, it is vital to treat your womb and entire body as sacred. Your womb is a temple—a vessel that holds your creative, sensual, and spiritual energy. By honoring its sacredness, you invite in only that which nurtures and respects you. This includes being mindful of who you allow into this sacred space. Engaging in unmindful or disconnected intimacy can leave emotional and energetic imprints that disrupt your inner balance. Take your time to decide who you will let into your sacred temple. This is an act of self-respect and self-love, rooted in recognizing your worth and honoring your boundaries.

When you approach intimacy with intention and clarity, you cultivate a deeper connection with yourself and your partner, transforming intimacy into a sacred, empowering, and mutually nurturing experience. This mindful connection reinforces the creative and sexual energy within you, enabling you to experience intimacy in a way that aligns with your values and enhances your wholeness.

A Story of Healing: The Talented Musician

One example that illustrates this journey is the story of a talented musician who faced immense trauma after being raped. Despite her incredible talent and passion for music, she found herself unable to fully connect with her creative energy. Her music, once a source of joy and expression, became stifled. The trauma she experienced had created energetic and emotional blocks within her womb space, leaving her disconnected from her creative essence. It was only when she committed to the process of womb healing—facing and releasing her trauma, working through layers of shame, and reclaiming her sensuality—that she experienced a profound shift. Her creative energy flowed once more, and her music took on a depth and authenticity that touched the hearts of many. Her story is a testament to the power of womb healing in restoring both creativity and self-expression.

Reclaiming Creative and Sexual Energy

Reclaiming our creative and sexual energy is an act of empowerment—a way to reconnect with the fullness of our being and to live from a place of authenticity and joy. By healing the womb, we honor the stories, wounds, and potential carried within, transforming blocks into gateways for self-discovery and self-expression.

Practices to Release Shame or Guilt and Reconnect with the Body's Pleasure Pathways

Releasing shame and guilt around sexuality is an essential part of reconnecting with the body's natural pleasure pathways. These practices are designed to help you let go of limiting beliefs around sexuality, embrace your sensual nature, and reclaim your creative, joyful self.

1. Body Awareness Meditation:

Begin by finding a quiet space where you can be undisturbed. Close your eyes and bring your awareness to your body, starting from the top of your head and gradually moving down to your toes.

As you scan your body, allow yourself to notice any areas where you feel tension, numbness, or resistance. These areas may carry unprocessed emotions or beliefs about shame, guilt, or unworthiness.

Gently breathe into each area, imagining each breath as a warm, golden light that softens and releases tension. Affirm to yourself that it's safe to feel pleasure and connect with your body.

2.Sacral Chakra Activation with Breathwork:

Sit comfortably, placing your hands over your lower abdomen. Focus on your sacral chakra, the energy center associated with creativity, sensuality, and emotion.

Begin deep belly breathing, visualizing an orange light expanding with each inhale and filling the entire lower abdomen.

With each exhale, release any stored guilt, shame, or tension around sexuality or creativity. Affirm that you are freeing yourself from any negative beliefs and making space for pleasure and creative flow.

3.Sensory Awakening Exercise:

Engage in an activity that stimulates one or more of your senses in a mindful way, such as savoring a piece of chocolate, feeling the warmth of the sun on your skin, or listening to your favorite music.

As you engage, allow yourself to fully experience each sensation without judgment. Notice any feelings of discomfort or resistance that arise and gently release them.

This exercise helps to reawaken the pleasure pathways in the body, allowing you to experience life's sensations fully and without shame.

4.Mirror Work for Body Acceptance:

Stand in front of a mirror and look at your body with kindness and appreciation. Begin by making eye contact with yourself, then let your gaze travel over your entire body. Speak words of love and acceptance to yourself. If it feels challenging, start with simple affirmations like, *"I love my body,"* or *"I honor my sensuality and creativity."* This practice helps to break down feelings of shame and builds a positive relationship with your body.

5.Creative Expression Ritual:

Choose a creative activity that feels natural to you, such as painting, writing, dancing, or singing. Before beginning, set an intention to let go of self-judgment and simply enjoy the process.

Engage in this activity without focusing on the end result. Allow yourself to be playful, expressive, and free.

This ritual is a way to connect with your creative energy, releasing the pressure to perform or produce and focusing instead on self-expression as an act of empowerment.

Journaling Prompts and Affirmations for Embracing Creativity and Sexuality

Using journaling prompts can be a powerful way to explore your inner beliefs about creativity and sexuality and to release any limitations that keep you from embracing these aspects of yourself. Here are some prompts to guide your exploration:

Journaling Prompts

1. What beliefs or messages about sexuality did I learn growing up? How have these beliefs influenced how I feel about my body and sensuality?

2. When do I feel most connected to my creative energy? What activities or situations make me feel fully alive and inspired?

3. Are there any areas in my life where I feel blocked creatively or sensually? What might be contributing to this feeling, and how can I begin to release it?

4. How would it feel to live without shame or guilt around my sexuality and creativity?

Describe what a day in this life would look and feel like.

5. What aspects of my sensuality and creativity do I find most empowering? How can I cultivate these aspects more fully in my daily life?

Affirmations for Creativity and Sexuality

Affirmations are a powerful tool for reprogramming the subconscious mind, helping to shift limiting beliefs and open yourself up to new possibilities. Here are some affirmations to support your journey of reconnecting with your creative and sexual energy:

"I am worthy of pleasure, joy, and creative expression."

"I release all shame and guilt surrounding my sexuality and embrace my sensual nature."

"My body is a sacred vessel of life, creativity, and love."

"I trust my intuition and allow my inner wisdom to guide my creative and sensual expression."

"I honor my body and celebrate its capacity for pleasure and creativity."

Repeat these affirmations daily, ideally in a space where you feel comfortable and undisturbed. You may also wish to incorporate them into your meditation practice, saying them quietly to yourself while placing your hands on your lower abdomen, symbolizing your connection with your womb.

Summary: Chapter 8

Reconnecting with your creative and sexual energy is a journey of self-discovery and empowerment. By releasing shame and guilt, you free yourself to experience life more fully, savoring its beauty, joy, and potential. Your womb is the sacred space where creativity and sensuality unite, offering a gateway to your inner strength and wisdom. Embracing this connection brings a renewed sense of purpose, vitality, and self-love, reminding you that you are a creator in every sense of the word.

Through these practices and affirmations, you are reclaiming the right to feel pleasure, express your creativity, and live authentically. As you journey deeper into womb healing, may you continue to honor your body, your spirit, and the creative power that flows through you. Let this reconnection to your sacred energy be a source of inspiration, empowerment, and profound joy.

Chapter 9: Womb Healing Practices for Physical Wellness

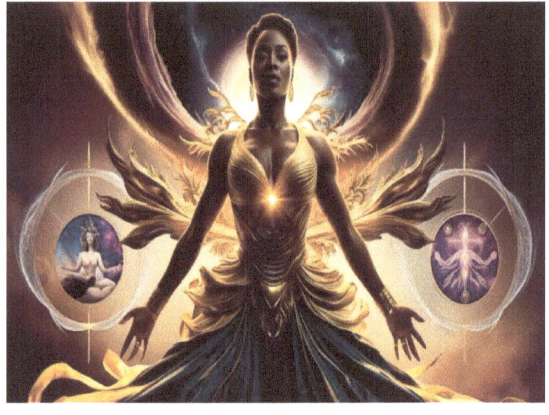

To achieve true wellness in the womb, we must address not only the emotional and energetic layers but also the physical aspects that contribute to its health. The womb is sensitive to what we consume, our lifestyle habits, and the daily stresses we experience. By adopting supportive practices—such as nourishing foods, gentle herbal remedies, and consistent self-care rituals—we create an environment in which our womb can thrive. This chapter will guide you through physical wellness practices that nurture, balance, and heal your womb, while also honoring its emotional, spiritual, and generational dimensions.

Lifestyle and Nutritional Practices for Womb Health

A balanced diet and lifestyle are foundational to womb health. Our food choices, level of physical activity, and daily routines impact our hormonal balance, inflammation levels, and overall reproductive health. It is essential to recognize that physical health practices can also influence our emotional and spiritual well-being, creating a holistic approach to womb healing. Here are key lifestyle and nutritional practices to support the womb.

1. Adopt an Anti-Inflammatory Diet:

Chronic inflammation can contribute to conditions like PCOS, endometriosis, and fibroids. An anti-inflammatory diet helps manage inflammation and reduce pain, making it a valuable approach for womb health.

Foods to Include: Fresh fruits (berries, oranges, cherries), vegetables (spinach, kale, broccoli), nuts, seeds, fatty fish (salmon, sardines), and healthy fats (olive oil, avocado).

Foods to Avoid: Refined sugars, processed foods, and trans fats, as well as excessive red meat and dairy, which can aggravate inflammation.

2. Focus on Hormone-Balancing Foods:

Hormonal balance is essential for womb health, especially for conditions like PCOS and fibroids. Certain foods help regulate estrogen and progesterone, the key hormones governing the menstrual cycle.

Cruciferous Vegetables: Vegetables like broccoli, cauliflower, and Brussels sprouts contain compounds that support estrogen metabolism.

Fiber-Rich Foods: High-fiber foods, such as legumes, whole grains, and leafy greens, help remove excess estrogen from the body.

Healthy Fats: Omega-3 fatty acids, found in walnuts, flaxseeds, and fish, are essential for hormone production and can reduce inflammation.

3. Maintain Regular Physical Activity: Regular movement encourages blood flow to the womb and pelvic area, supporting optimal function. Gentle exercises like walking, swimming, and yoga help maintain a healthy weight, reduce inflammation, and balance hormones.

Yoga for Womb Health: Yoga postures such as the goddess pose, child's pose, and hip openers (like pigeon pose) encourage circulation and relaxation in the pelvic region, relieving tension and balancing energy.

Physical activity also helps release stored tension, promoting emotional clarity and connecting mind and body.

4. Stay Hydrated:

Hydration is vital for every bodily function, including hormonal balance and waste removal. Drinking adequate water supports the kidneys and liver, which help remove excess hormones and toxins that could otherwise accumulate in the womb.

Consider infusing water with herbs like mint or lemon for additional detoxifying effects, and recognize that proper hydration also supports emotional balance and mental clarity.

5. Herbal Remedies, Supplements, and Self-Care Techniques for Womb Health

Natural remedies, when combined with a balanced lifestyle, can provide additional support to the womb, easing symptoms and promoting overall wellness. Here are specific herbal remedies, supplements, and self-care techniques that can nourish and support the womb.

Red Raspberry Leaf: Known as the "woman's herb," red raspberry leaf is high in nutrients that support the uterus, ease menstrual cramps, and tone the uterine muscles.

Chasteberry (Vitex): Chasteberry can help regulate hormonal imbalances, particularly for conditions like PMS and PCOS, by supporting progesterone levels.

Ashwagandha: An adaptogen that reduces stress and supports hormonal balance, ashwagandha can be beneficial for overall reproductive health.

Dong Quai: Often used in traditional Chinese medicine, dong quai helps improve circulation to the pelvic area and reduce menstrual pain. It is best used under professional guidance, as it may not be suitable for all women.

6. Supplements for Womb Health:

Magnesium: Known for its muscle-relaxing properties, magnesium can reduce menstrual cramps and support adrenal health, which in turn affects hormonal balance.

Zinc: Zinc is essential for immune health and hormonal function, and it plays a role in reproductive health. Foods high in zinc include pumpkin seeds, lentils, and chickpeas.

B Vitamins: Particularly B6 and B12, these vitamins support liver detoxification, helping to regulate hormone levels and reduce symptoms like PMS and bloating.

7. Self-Care Techniques:

Castor Oil Packs: Applying castor oil packs over the lower abdomen promotes circulation, reduces inflammation, and supports lymphatic drainage. Castor oil packs are often used for conditions like fibroids, cysts, and endometriosis.

Warm Compresses: A simple warm compress applied to the lower abdomen can soothe cramps, relax muscles, and ease discomfort during menstruation.

Self-Massage: Gently massaging the abdomen in a clockwise direction helps improve blood flow to the womb, relieve tension, and enhance relaxation.

8. Limit Environmental Toxins:

Hormone disruptors, often found in plastics, cosmetics, and cleaning products, can interfere with natural hormone balance. Choose natural or organic alternatives when possible and avoid plastics, especially for food storage, to reduce your exposure to these chemicals.

Guided Physical Healing Meditation for the Womb

This meditation is designed to release physical tension, reduce pain, and restore harmony to the womb. Practicing this meditation regularly can help deepen your connection with your womb, release physical and emotional blockages, and support healing.

Preparation:

➢ Find a quiet, comfortable space where you won't be disturbed.

➢ Lie down with your knees bent or in a seated position with your spine straight.

Meditation Steps:
Centering Breath:
Begin by taking slow, deep breaths, inhaling through your nose and exhaling

gently through your mouth. Allow each breath to relax your body and bring your awareness inward.

Focus on your womb area, feeling it rise gently with each inhale and settle with each exhale.

Visualizing Warm Light:

Imagine a warm, gentle light glowing in the center of your womb, illuminating it with healing energy. See this light as golden or soft pink—whatever color feels soothing to you.

With each inhale, feel this light expanding, filling your entire womb area with warmth and comfort. With each exhale, imagine any tension or discomfort dissolving and leaving your body.

Releasing Physical Tension:

Scan your womb area and notice any areas that feel tight, tense, or uncomfortable.

Bring your awareness to these areas without judgment, simply observing them. As you exhale, visualize these areas softening, allowing any discomfort to dissipate with each breath. If it feels right, place your hands over your lower abdomen to provide comforting support.

Affirming Healing:

Silently or out loud, repeat gentle affirmations such as:

"My womb is a place of peace and wellness."

"I release all pain and tension from my womb."

"My body supports me, and I honor its wisdom."

Let each affirmation infuse your womb with positive, healing energy, reinforcing the idea of balance and harmony within.

Envisioning Wholeness:

Now, visualize your womb as a healthy, radiant center within your body, free from pain and filled with vibrant energy. Imagine this energy flowing freely through your body, connecting with your heart, mind, and soul. Feel yourself as whole, complete, and empowered, honoring the sacredness of your womb.

Closing the Meditation:

Take a few more deep breaths, gently bringing your awareness back to the present moment.

When you feel ready, open your eyes, feeling grounded and at peace.

Summary: Chapter 9

The womb is a sacred and powerful center within the female body, capable of creation, intuition, and transformation. By supporting womb health through nourishing foods, herbal remedies, and gentle self-care practices, we honor this vital part of ourselves. The physical healing meditation serves as a practice of self-love and connection, helping you release tension and infuse your womb with positive energy. Embracing these womb-healing practices cultivates not only physical wellness but also a deeper appreciation of your body's wisdom and strength.

In nurturing the womb, we nurture ourselves. This journey of physical wellness for the womb is an essential step in reclaiming your health, creativity, and inner harmony, allowing you to live more fully in alignment with your true self.

Chapter 10: Living with the Empowered Womb

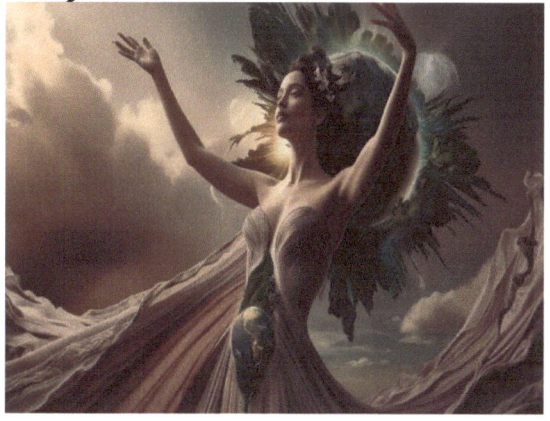

The journey of womb healing is transformative, guiding women to release inherited trauma, reclaim self-worth, and reconnect with their deepest source of wisdom and creativity. Through each step, we have uncovered layers of emotional and energetic blockages, liberated ourselves from societal and generational patterns, and opened the way for authentic self-expression. By reconnecting with the womb, we have accessed a source of intuition, inner power, and nurturing energy that empowers us to live fully.

Living with an empowered womb is an ongoing journey, one that requires commitment and a conscious connection to this center of wisdom. It means honoring the feminine essence within us and embodying this energy in all areas of our lives. When we are connected to our womb space, we live with greater alignment, purpose, and joy, grounded in the knowledge that we carry the power to create, heal, and transform.

Embodying Empowered Feminine Energy in Daily Life

As we complete this journey of womb healing, it is essential to integrate this empowered energy into our daily lives, allowing it to guide our actions, relationships, and choices. Here are ways to embody this renewed sense of feminine power.

1. In Relationships:

An empowered womb brings clarity, helping us set healthy boundaries and communicate authentically. When we are in touch with this center, we relate to others from a place of completeness and wholeness, rather than seeking external validation. Honor the needs of your womb by fostering relationships that respect your energy and well-being.

Practice openness, empathy, and emotional expression with those you trust. This allows you to share your empowered feminine energy with others in a way that is nurturing, compassionate, and respectful.

2. In Work and Creativity:

Embrace the womb as a source of creative inspiration and ideas. Whether your work involves art, leadership, or problem-solving, trust the intuitive insights and innovative ideas that emerge from this space. Let your creativity flow freely, unbound by limitations or expectations.

In moments of self-doubt, return to your womb space, reconnecting with its innate power and grounding energy. This practice will remind you of your ability to create, nurture, and bring meaningful contributions to the world.

3. In Self-Care and Personal Growth:

Prioritize self-care practices that honor your feminine energy, such as regular meditation, gentle movement, and nourishing foods. Remember that living with an empowered womb involves tending to the physical, emotional, and spiritual aspects of yourself with compassion.

Continue exploring inner healing through journaling, energy work, or creative expression. Make time to listen to your inner voice and honor the emotions and insights that arise from this space.

4. In Intimacy and Sensuality:

Embrace your sensuality as a natural extension of your womb's energy. Living with an empowered womb means embracing your body, enjoying physical experiences, and connecting with your senses. Allow yourself to experience intimacy and pleasure without guilt or shame, and honor your body's wisdom in all aspects of your life.

Breaking the Cycle of Trauma and Releasing Our Children from Epigenetic Effects

Living with an empowered womb is also about breaking generational cycles of trauma and creating a new legacy for future generations. By healing the wounds carried within our wombs, we release our children from the burden of inherited trauma and allow them to grow without the weight of unprocessed pain. Epigenetic research shows that trauma experienced by one generation can affect the genetic expression of subsequent generations, but healing can alter this legacy. As we release these imprints, we open the door for our children to live more freely, authentically, and joyfully.

Healing Through Connection and Conscious Parenting: As mothers, mentors, or nurturers, we have the opportunity to model healthy, empowered relationships with ourselves and our bodies. This connection provides our children with a foundation of self-worth, empathy, and resilience.

Breaking Patterns of Suppression: By embracing our empowered feminine energy, we teach the next generation to honor their emotions, boundaries, and intuitive wisdom.

We give them permission to break free from societal narratives that seek to diminish their value or silence their voices.

A Closing Ritual for Honoring the Empowered Womb

To celebrate this journey of transformation and reaffirm your commitment to honoring the sacred womb, here is a closing ritual designed to acknowledge your progress, embrace your empowered feminine energy, and continue the connection with this center of wisdom.

Womb Empowerment Ritual

Preparation:

➢ Find a quiet, comfortable space where

you won't be disturbed. Light a candle or some incense to create a peaceful, sacred atmosphere. Have a journal and pen nearby to capture any insights that arise.

Step 1: Grounding and Centering

Begin by sitting or lying down comfortably. Close your eyes and take a few deep breaths, feeling the air fill your lungs and release any tension in your body.

Visualize roots growing from your feet, connecting you to the earth. Feel the grounding energy of the earth flowing up into your body, anchoring you in the present moment.

Step 2: Connecting to the Womb

Place your hands gently over your lower abdomen, tuning into your womb space. Imagine a warm, gentle light radiating from within, filling your hands and your entire abdomen with a comforting glow.

As you breathe, visualize this light expanding, illuminating your womb and connecting you to the journey you've been on—the release, the healing, and the transformation.

Step 3: Reflect on Your Journey
Take a moment to reflect on the experiences, insights, and emotional releases you've had during this journey. Acknowledge the changes you've made, the pain you've let go, and the strength you've gained.
Silently express gratitude to your womb for being your guide and for the wisdom it holds. Feel a sense of pride for the growth and empowerment you have achieved.

Step 4: Affirmations of Empowerment
Silently or aloud, repeat affirmations that reinforce your commitment to honoring your womb and embracing your feminine power:

"I honor my womb as a sacred center of creation, intuition, and wisdom."

"I release all past pain and embrace my empowered feminine energy."

"I am whole, complete, and connected to my sacred feminine essence."

"I trust the wisdom of my womb to guide me in all areas of my life."

Step 5: Setting an Intention for the Future

In your journal, write a few sentences describing how you intend to live with an empowered womb going forward. This could be a commitment to self-care, an intention to nurture creativity, or a goal to cultivate loving relationships. Let this intention serve as a guiding light in the days and weeks to come.

Step 6: Seal the Ritual

Place your hands over your womb once more and visualize a golden light encircling it, like a protective shield of love and strength.

When you feel ready, slowly open your eyes. Take a few moments to ground yourself in the present moment and close the ritual by extinguishing the candle, symbolizing a fresh start and a commitment to your empowered self.

Summary: Chapter 10

Living with an empowered womb is an invitation to fully inhabit your feminine power, to honor your intuition, and to embrace a life that is in harmony with your true self. This journey of womb healing has allowed you to reconnect with your innate wisdom, creativity, and strength. By continuing to nurture this connection, you not only transform your own life but also contribute to the collective healing of feminine energy and the creation of a society where men and women stand together in balance, mutual respect, and shared purpose.

The empowered womb is a source of love, wisdom, and resilience that guides you to live authentically, joyfully, and compassionately. As you move forward, trust the messages from this sacred space, honor the journey you've taken, and embrace the limitless potential that lies within you. Together, we can create a world of harmony and wholeness for ourselves and future generations.

Bonus Section: Practical Resources and Tools for Ongoing Womb Healing

This bonus section provides practical resources to support your ongoing womb healing journey. These tools and practices are designed to help you cultivate a daily or weekly routine of nurturing, reflection, and connection with your womb space. Remember, womb healing is a process, and consistency in these practices can bring profound shifts in your emotional, physical, and spiritual well-being.

1. Affirmations, Meditations, and Rituals for Womb Healing

Affirmations for Womb Healing

Affirmations help reprogram limiting beliefs and reinforce positive self-worth. Repeat these affirmations daily, especially when you feel disconnected or in need of grounding:

➢ "I am connected to the wisdom of my womb and honor its sacred power."

➢ "I release all inherited pain and embrace my feminine strength."

➢ "My womb is a source of creativity, intuition, and healing."

➢ "I am worthy of love, joy, and fulfillment."

➢ "I nurture myself with compassion and embrace my emotions fully."

➢ "I honor the strength of my ancestors and release their pain with love."

➢ "My womb is a source of joy, creativity, and sacred connection."

➢ "I reclaim my body and my power as my own."

Choose a few affirmations that resonate deeply with you. Write them on sticky notes, journal them, or say them aloud each morning.

Meditations for Womb Healing

Meditation is a powerful tool for connecting with your womb and accessing the deep emotions and wisdom stored within. Here's a simple meditation practice to get started:

Find a Quiet Space: Sit or lie down comfortably. Close your eyes and take a few deep breaths, letting go of any tension.

Focus on Your Womb: Bring your awareness to your lower abdomen, just below the navel. Imagine a warm, soft light growing in this area, like a small, nurturing sun.

1. **Breathe into the Womb**: With each inhale, feel this light expanding, filling your womb with warmth and comfort. With each exhale, imagine any tension, pain, or negative energy gently leaving your body.

2. **Ancestral Connection Visualization**: Imagine yourself in a circle with your female ancestors, sharing their wisdom and releasing their pain, creating a lineage of healing.

3. **Set an Intention**: Silently set an intention, such as *"I am open to healing and releasing all that no longer serves me."*

4. **Visualization for Emotional Release**: Envision placing all burdens, traumas, and negative beliefs into a symbolic vessel in your womb, and then releasing it into the earth or transforming it with light.

5. **Listen and Reflect**: Spend a few minutes simply feeling the presence of your womb, allowing any emotions, insights, or memories to surface. Accept whatever arises without judgment.

6. **Close with Gratitude**: When you're ready, slowly bring your awareness back to the room. Place your hands on your womb and silently express gratitude for this connection and the wisdom within.

Rituals for Womb Healing

Creating rituals for womb healing adds depth and meaning to the practice. Here are a few you can try.

1. **Moon Ritual**: Align your womb healing rituals with the moon cycle.

New Moon Womb Healing Circle: Gather with other women (in-person or virtually) to set collective intentions for healing, share stories, and engage in a group meditation. This promotes the power of communal healing and reinforces the connection to cyclical energies.

Full Moon Release Ceremony: Engage in a ritual to release any accumulated emotions, beliefs, or traumas. This can involve writing down what you're ready to let go of and symbolically burning the paper or burying it in the earth.

2. **Warm Compress with Essential Oils**: Apply a warm compress to your lower abdomen with a few drops of essential oils like clary sage, rose, or lavender. As you place the compress on your womb, breathe deeply and visualize warmth and healing energy infusing your womb space.

3. **Journaling Ritual**: At the end of each week, take a few moments to journal about your emotions, experiences, and any shifts you noticed in your body. Writing down your reflections is a way of honoring your

journey and setting intentions for continued healing.

Recommended Books, Articles, Courses, and Communities for Further Exploration

Books

Womb Awakening: Initiatory Wisdom from the Creatrix of All Life by Azra Bertrand and Seren Bertrand – A mystical exploration of the womb's spiritual power.

Sacred Woman: A Guide to Healing the Feminine Body, Mind, and Spirit by Queen Afua – Offers guidance on feminine healing rituals, rooted in African spiritual traditions.

The Wild Feminine: Finding Power, Spirit, and Joy in the Female Body by Tami Lynn Kent

Wild Power: Discover the Magic of Your Menstrual Cycle and Awaken the Feminine Path to Power by Alexandra Pope and Sjanie Hugo Wurlitzer – Explores the power of the menstrual cycle as a gateway to personal empowerment.

Heal Your Womb, Heal Your Life: A Guide for Healing from Fibroids and Other Womb Dis-Ease by Diane M. Speier

The Body Keeps the Score: Brain, Mind, and Body in the Healing of Trauma by Bessel van der Kolk – This book explores the deep connection between trauma and physical symptoms, providing valuable insights for womb healing.

Women Who Run With the Wolves by Clarissa Pinkola Estés – A powerful exploration of feminine archetypes and the reclaiming of wild, untamed energy within.

Articles

"Epigenetic Mechanisms in the Inheritance of Generational Trauma" by Rachel Yehuda and Amy E. Bierer, *Biological Psychiatry*

"The Role of Emotions in Physical Health: Exploring the Mind-Body Connection" by Candace Pert, *Molecules of Emotion*

"Reclaiming the Feminine Power Within" by Marion Woodman, exploring the power of the feminine archetype and its effects on personal healing.

Courses

The Wellbeing Sanctuary (DecodeYou®)

– Explore workshops or courses that integrate subconscious reprogramming, ancestral healing, and womb-centered therapies.

Red School's Menstruality Training – A

course that guides women through reconnecting with the natural cycles of their bodies, with emphasis on healing and personal empowerment.

Womb Awakening Practitioner Training – A program focused on shamanic and mystical womb healing practices for both personal and professional development.

Trauma-Informed Yoga and Breathwork Courses: These focus on connecting with the body, especially the pelvic and womb areas, in a safe and gentle way to release trauma.

Holistic Nutrition for Reproductive Health: Programs that focus on dietary and lifestyle practices to support hormonal balance and womb wellness

Communities

The Wild Feminine Community – An online network led by Tami Lynn Kent, where women share stories, practices, and experiences of womb-centered healing.

Women's Circles and Red Tents – Many communities offer Red Tent gatherings or women's circles, safe spaces for sharing experiences, supporting each other, and engaging in collective healing.

Social Media Groups – Facebook and other social media platforms host groups dedicated to womb healing, menstrual health, and feminine empowerment, allowing women to connect and support each other's journeys.

Additional Tools and Practices for Womb Healing

Bodywork and Somatic Therapies:

I recommend therapies such as **abdominal massage**, **pelvic floor therapy**, or **craniosacral therapy**, which can help release physical and energetic blockages in the womb area.

Somatic experiencing as a method to release trauma stored in the body, with a focus on the pelvic and womb areas.

Art and Creative Expression:

I suggest engaging in creative expression, such as **painting, writing, or crafting**, that focuses on the womb's energy. Art can be a powerful way to process and transform emotions.

4. A Sample Daily or Weekly Routine for Maintaining Womb Health and Emotional Balance

This sample routine provides a balanced structure of daily and weekly practices to nurture your womb health and maintain emotional balance. Adjust it as needed to suit your schedule and needs.

Daily Routine

Morning: Begin your day with a few affirmations as you wake up. Set a positive intention to stay connected with your womb and embrace your feminine energy.

Breathwork: Spend 5–10 minutes focusing on deep belly breathing, bringing awareness to your womb with each breath.

Body Movement: Incorporate gentle yoga, especially poses that open the hips and stretch the lower abdomen, such as Pigeon Pose, Child's Pose, and Butterfly Pose.

This helps to stimulate circulation and energy flow around the womb.

Reflection: Before bed, place your hands over your womb and take a few moments to breathe deeply and reflect on your day. Acknowledge any emotions or sensations that came up, and release any tension or stress from your womb space.

Weekly Routine

Meditation Practice: Dedicate 15–20 minutes once a week to a focused womb meditation (such as the one described earlier), allowing time to connect deeply with your womb and release any accumulated emotions.

Self-Care Ritual: Take a warm bath with Epsom salts and a few drops of essential oils like clary sage or rose, which help balance hormones and soothe the womb area. Allow yourself to relax and meditate on self-love.

Journaling: Choose one day each week to journal about any changes or insights you noticed in your womb health, emotions, or creative energy. Use this time to reflect on any patterns you're noticing and set intentions for the following week.

Engage with a Community: Connect with a women's circle, support group, or online community to share your experiences and gather inspiration. Engaging with others on a similar path offers support and insight that enriches your healing journey.

Closing Thoughts

Ongoing womb healing requires a commitment to nurturing, reflection, and self-care. By integrating affirmations, meditations, rituals, and connecting with a community of like-minded women, you create a strong foundation for emotional and physical well-being. On one hand, this journey is deeply personal, and each practice can be tailored to what feels right for you. Through these resources and practices, you can maintain a harmonious relationship with your womb, honoring its sacred energy as a source of strength, creativity, and wisdom. On the other hand, it is a collective movement that has the power to transform society. When women heal their wombs, they not only reclaim their own power but also contribute to the healing of generational trauma, the rebalancing of masculine and feminine energies, and the creation of a society where men and women stand in harmony—neither in dominance nor in submission, but as equal partners in the journey of life.

Appendices

1. Glossary of Terms

This glossary provides definitions for key terms used throughout the book, offering readers clarity on concepts related to womb healing, energy, and transformation.

Sacral Energy: Energy located in the sacral chakra, the energy center just below the navel. Sacral energy governs creativity, sexuality, pleasure, and emotional expression. It connects us with our sense of self, emotions, and sensuality.

Ancestral Healing: A process of addressing unresolved emotional and psychological issues passed down from previous generations. Ancestral healing involves recognizing and releasing inherited patterns, beliefs, and traumas that may unconsciously influence one's present life.

Subconscious Reprogramming: Techniques used to identify and change limiting beliefs and negative thought patterns stored in the subconscious mind. Subconscious reprogramming often involves visualization, affirmations, and meditative practices to replace old beliefs with empowering new ones.

Generational Trauma: Emotional and psychological trauma that is passed down from one generation to the next, often stemming from unresolved experiences of previous generations. Generational trauma can manifest as emotional pain, limiting beliefs, or fears.

Energetic Imprints: Emotional or psychological experiences that are stored in the body, particularly in energy centers like the womb or sacral chakra. These imprints can influence behavior, emotional responses, and physical health.

Sacral Chakra(Swadhisthana): The second chakra, located in the lower abdomen, associated with creativity, sexuality, emotional expression, and pleasure. When balanced, the sacral chakra supports emotional well-being and a healthy connection to one's desires and relationships.

Inner Child Healing: A therapeutic process focused on reconnecting with and nurturing the inner child—the part of us that holds childhood experiences, memories, and feelings. Inner child healing addresses unmet emotional needs and resolves patterns formed during early life.

Epigenetics: The study of changes in gene expression caused by environmental factors rather than alterations in the DNA sequence. Epigenetics shows how trauma or stress in one generation can affect genetic expression in subsequent generations.

Mind-Body Connection: The understanding that mental and emotional states can impact physical health. The mind-body connection is foundational in holistic healing, acknowledging that unresolved emotional pain can manifest as physical symptoms.

Goddess Archetype: In psychology and spirituality, the goddess archetype represents aspects of the feminine psyche, including wisdom, nurturing, intuition, and power. Connecting with goddess archetypes can inspire and empower women to embrace their feminine strengths.

Somatic Healing: A therapeutic approach focused on the body to release stored trauma and emotions. Somatic healing techniques, such as breathwork and body awareness practices, help individuals process and release trauma held in the body.

Sacred Feminine: The concept of the divine feminine energy within each individual, encompassing qualities like intuition, compassion, creation, and nurturing. Sacred feminine energy is often associated with the womb and feminine power.

Womb Wisdom: The intuitive knowledge and guidance that comes from connecting deeply with the womb, encompassing creativity, instinctual awareness, and emotional intelligence.

Yoni: A term from Sanskrit often used to describe the vulva and womb, symbolizing feminine power, creativity, and sacred space.

Reproductive Sovereignty: The concept of reclaiming control and autonomy over one's reproductive health, decisions, and well-being.

Sacred Feminine Circles: Gatherings of women for support, healing, and empowerment, often focused on nurturing feminine energy and sharing personal journeys.

List of Practices and Exercises

This section provides a quick reference for practices and exercises outlined in each chapter, allowing readers to easily revisit and incorporate them into their daily routines.

Chapter 1: Understanding the Whispers of the Womb

Womb Connection Meditation: A practice to connect with the womb as an energy center, focusing on the womb's role in creativity and intuition.

Sacral Chakra Balancing Visualization: A guided visualization to balance and cleanse the sacral chakra, supporting emotional and physical health.

Chapter 2: The Ancestral Imprints in the Womb

Ancestral Reflection Exercise: Journaling prompts and reflective questions to identify inherited beliefs and generational patterns.

Ancestral Release Meditation: A meditation for recognizing and releasing inherited emotional imprints from previous generations.

Chapter 3: Recognizing Physical Manifestations of Womb Imbalances

Body Scan for Womb Awareness: A mindfulness practice for recognizing and understanding physical sensations or discomfort in the womb area.

Emotion Mapping Exercise: An exercise to link physical symptoms with emotional states, identifying connections between emotional pain and physical manifestations.

Chapter 4: Releasing Emotional Trauma Stored in the Womb

Guided Womb Healing Meditation: A meditation focused on releasing stored trauma, addressing feelings of shame, grief, or unworthiness.

Journaling for Emotional Release: Prompts to help identify and process unexpressed emotions held in the womb.

Chapter 5: Reclaiming Your Feminine Power Through Subconscious Reprogramming

Limiting Belief Identification Exercise: A practice to identify subconscious beliefs and replace them with empowering thoughts.

Visualization for Self-Worth: A visualization exercise to affirm and reinforce feelings of self-worth and feminine power.

Chapter 6: Healing Generational Inadequacies and Breaking Cycles

Generational Dialogue Exercise: A meditation or visualization practice to connect with ancestors and release generational inadequacies.

Affirmations for Generational Healing: Positive affirmations to support the healing of inherited emotional patterns.

Chapter 7: Integrating Womb Healing with Energy Practices

Reiki for Womb Healing: Steps for a simple Reiki practice focused on the womb.

Sacral Chakra Breathing: Breathwork to release blockages in the sacral chakra, enhancing emotional and energetic flow.

Chapter 8: Reconnecting with Creative and Sexual Energy

Creative Expression Exercise: A guided practice to channel sacral energy into creative pursuits.

Sensual Awareness Meditation: A meditation to embrace and reconnect with the body's pleasure pathways, fostering self-love.

Chapter 9: Womb Healing Practices for Physical Wellness

Nutrition for Womb Health: Guidelines on anti-inflammatory foods and herbs that support hormonal balance and reproductive health.

Physical Womb Healing Meditation: A focused meditation for physical relief and nurturing of the womb area.

Chapter 10: Living with the Empowered Womb

Empowered Self-Ritual: A closing ritual to honor the womb and reinforce a commitment to self-love, creative expression, and nurturing.

Daily Affirmations for Womb Healing: A collection of affirmations to incorporate into daily life, supporting ongoing healing and empowerment.

Conclusion: Embracing a Life of Wholeness and Worth

For me, this journey has been deeply personal and transformative. As a woman, I have navigated the myriad emotional challenges women face—grappling with self-worth, societal expectations, health struggles, and the quest to reclaim a sense of self. These experiences have not only shaped who I am but have guided me in finding solutions for my clients. My own journey, intertwined with the stories of countless women I have worked with, has illuminated a path of healing, resilience, and empowerment. This is why I feel so deeply called to write this book.

The purpose of this book is to bring awareness and make healing accessible to all women—those who have suffered silently, felt disconnected from their bodies, or struggled under societal expectations and inherited trauma. It serves as a guide, companion, and source of inspiration for every woman seeking to reconnect with her womb, her essence, and her power. It is a tool for breaking free from patterns of suppression, shame, and self-doubt, and for reclaiming the wholeness that is our birthright.

Through this book, I seek to illuminate the womb's sacredness—not merely as an organ, but as a center of profound wisdom, creativity, and healing. It is a call for women to step into their power by understanding and addressing the deeper layers of their existence—the subconscious patterns, generational imprints, societal narratives, and personal traumas that have shaped their lives. By offering practical tools, guided reflections, and wisdom drawn from my own journey and the journeys of my clients, this book provides a pathway to healing and transformation.

In its pages, I share not only personal stories but also the collective wisdom of generations of women and insights gained from years of working with clients. This book is for those who seek to break free from cycles of pain, shame, and suppression; it is a roadmap for reconnecting with the power, intuition, and joy that resides within each of us. My hope is that every woman who reads these pages will feel seen, understood, and empowered to embark on her own healing journey—knowing she is not alone and that deep transformation is within her reach.

My vision is to create a movement of empowered women—women who understand that healing the womb means healing themselves and, by extension, the world around them. It is a movement toward balance, harmony, and partnership with men—not rooted in dominance or submission but in mutual respect and shared strength. This book is my offering, my prayer, and my commitment to creating a world where women can thrive in their wholeness and share their unique light with the world. I hope it becomes a source of inspiration, healing, and empowerment for all who read it.

The journey of womb healing, a journey of reclaiming self-worth, creativity, and inner peace is an act of courage, one that calls us to trust in our own power and honor our unique path. As we heal, we not only change our relationship with ourselves but also with the world around us. We step into our lives with renewed confidence, expressing our creativity and emotions freely, and living with a sense of purpose that comes from within. We embody the wisdom of our ancestors, the strength of our experiences, and the beauty of our uniqueness.

I believe that womb healing is a path to self-discovery, wholeness, and empowerment. It allows us to break free from the stories and patterns that no longer serve us, to heal the wounds of the past, and to create a new legacy of strength, love, and authenticity. It is my sincere wish that this book serves as a source of light and inspiration—a guide that empowers women to step fully into their own power, nurture their inner sanctuary, and live lives of purpose, joy, and deep fulfillment.

If you feel inspired to explore more, have questions, or wish to share your reflections, I would be honored to connect with you. You can reach me at **info@yourwellbeingsanctuary.com** or

through my website at
https://qrco.de/bfeXJc.

Together, let us embark on this journey of healing and transformation, creating a world where every woman stands in her truth, honors her sacredness, and embodies the wholeness that is her birthright.

With love and gratitude,

Sarmistha Mitra.

About The Author

Sarmistha Mitra

Sarmistha Mitra is a master holistic counselor, thought leader, and philosopher with over a decade of experience exploring the intricate workings of the human mind.

She is the founder of The Wellbeing Sanctuary (https://qrco.de/bfeXJc) and the innovative mind-training model DecodeYou®: A Path to Self-Mastery. Her work aims to guide individuals toward unraveling subconscious patterns and healing trauma bonds by embracing both their inner strengths and vulnerabilities. Sarmistha is also the author of two Amazon bestselling books.
Whispers Of The Womb : Healing Generations and Reclaiming Feminine Power, is her third book, expanding her

exploration into the sacred feminine, ancestral healing, and energetic transformation. She is committed to bringing profound emotional freedom and healing to those who seek transformation, helping individuals understand the power of their subconscious to initiate lasting change.

Books By This Author

The Intricate Web of Trauma Bonding and Attachment

In The Intricate Web of Trauma Bonding, and Attachment, holistic psychologist Sarmistha Mitra unravels the complex dynamics of trauma bonds through the lenses of both science and metaphysics. This book offers readers a deep understanding of how neurochemical processes like the release of endorphins can keep individuals stuck in cycles of pain and intermittent relief in relationships. By blending this scientific insight with metaphysical principles such as yin-yang energy balance and karmic healing, Mitra provides a holistic approach to emotional liberation.

Through exploring the evolutionary role of

social bonds, Mitra explains why we are biologically wired to maintain attachments—even toxic ones—and how trauma bonding, reinforced by the brain's pain-relief system, mirrors addiction. She offers practical tools to break these destructive cycles by restoring emotional balance, reclaiming autonomy, and healing generational trauma.

Timeless Wisdfom : A Chronicle

Timeless Wisdom: A Chronicle is a profound tapestry woven with narratives that traverse the boundaries of time, culture, and consciousness. Through twelve deeply stirring stories, this book embarks on a journey that bridges the realms of past, present, and future. Each story reveals profound truths and touches the deepest recesses of the human heart, leaving an indelible mark on readers.

The book is divided into four intricate

sections, each designed to take readers on a transformative journey of self-discovery, reflection, and healing.

1. Inner Healing and Self-Rediscovery
The first section invites readers to confront their innermost shadows and wounds. Through stories of characters facing loss, betrayal, and the weight of their past, readers are guided toward self-awareness and healing. These tales exemplify how we can reclaim our power by understanding and nurturing our truest selves. Each narrative emphasizes the power of forgiveness, self-compassion, and facing life's darkest moments with courage.

2. Ancestral Patterns and Karmic Cycles
Delving into the intricacies of inherited patterns and karmic ties, this section illuminates how our ancestors' choices

shape our present lives. Through evocative stories steeped in generational struggles and triumphs, readers gain insights into breaking free from self-limiting cycles. The tales reflect on the idea that every wound carries a lesson and a chance to rewrite destiny.

3. Archetypes and Symbolic Journeys
Drawing upon the power of archetypes and symbolism, these stories explore the timeless roles we embody in life's grand narrative. Readers meet healers, seekers, wisdom keepers, and warriors navigating inner and outer worlds. Through rich allegories and symbolic quests, the narratives offer new ways of seeing ourselves and others, igniting a deeper connection to our purpose and the universal truths that bind humanity.

4. Unconditional Love and Acceptance
The final section celebrates the transformative power of love in its purest form. These stories traverse the spectrum of human connection—parental bonds, friendships, soul partnerships, and self-love. Readers are guided through tales of compassion, redemption, and unconditional acceptance, showing how love heals and unites all.

Timeless Wisdom: A Chronicle is more than just a collection of stories; it is a spiritual guide, a philosophical reflection, and an emotional journey meant to resonate through lifetimes. Each story acts as a mirror, inviting readers to explore their own experiences, seek deeper truths, and ultimately, find peace within themselves and their relationships. This book promises to be a legacy of wisdom for generations to come, intricately weaving science, metaphysics, and spirituality in a poetic dance that echoes through time.

www.ingramcontent.com/pod-product-compliance
Lightning Source LLC
LaVergne TN
LVHW072012080526
838199LV00096B/643